Echocardiography

This book sets echocardiography within a routine clinical context. It aims to synthesise guidelines into a pragmatic clinical approach to real patients, providing a step-by-step guide to performing, reporting, and interpreting a study. We wrote it imagining we were the calm voice of a senior echocardiographer teaching a junior colleague. This edition has been extensively revised with an expansion of sections on acute, intensive care and emergency medicine. COVID-19 has necessitated limiting exposure of both patient and operator to infection and caused a huge increase in waiting lists. This has sharpened the debate over matching the level of scan to the clinical question and also highlights the importance of collaboration between clinicians and echocardiographers.

Key Features

- Expanded first chapter on levels of echocardiography
- New sections on COVID-19, cardio-oncology, multivalve disease, and specialist valve clinics
- Incorporation of new international guidelines, grading criteria, and normal data
- Guide to how cardiac CT and magnetic resonance can complement echocardiography
- Reformatted text and extra diagrams and tables to improve understanding

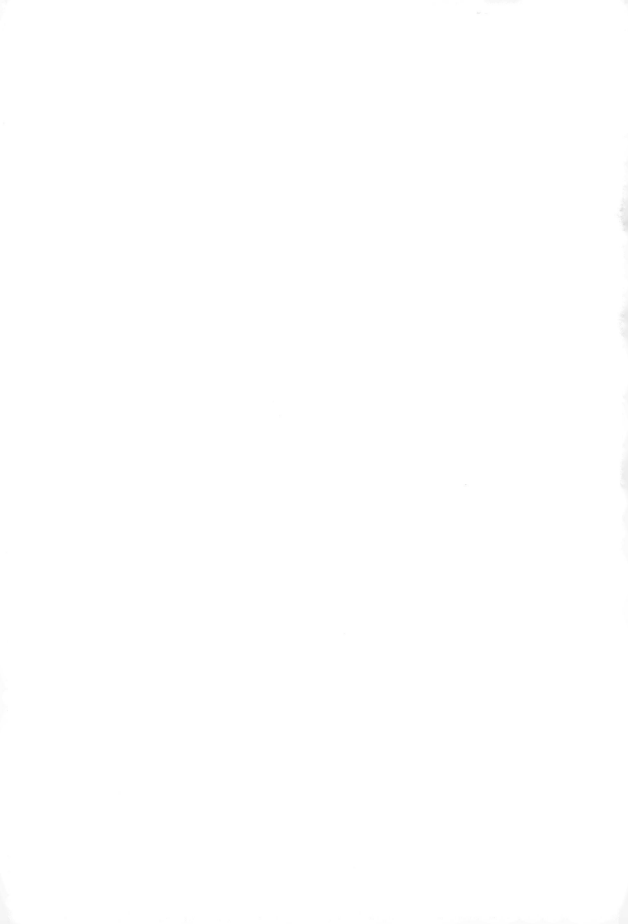

Echocardiography

A Practical Guide for Reporting and Interpretation

Fourth Edition

Camelia Demetrescu BSc, MSc, HSSE
Consultant Clinical Scientist in Cardiology
Guy's and St Thomas' Hospitals, London

Sandeep S Hothi MA, PhD, FRCP, FACC, FBSE, FESC
Consultant Cardiologist
Royal Wolverhampton NHS Trust
Honorary Senior Clinical Lecturer
University of Birmingham

John Chambers MD, FESC, FACC
Emeritus Professor of Clinical Cardiology
Guy's and St Thomas' Hospitals, London

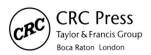

CRC Press
Taylor & Francis Group
Boca Raton London

CRC Press is an imprint of the
Taylor & Francis Group, an **informa** business

Fourth edition published 2024
by CRC Press
6000 Broken Sound Parkway NW, Suite 300, Boca Raton, FL 33487–2742

and by CRC Press
4 Park Square, Milton Park, Abingdon, Oxon, OX14 4RN

CRC Press is an imprint of Taylor & Francis Group, LLC

© 2024 Camelia Demetrescu, Sandeep S Hothi and John Chambers

ISBN: 978-1-032-15160-1 (hbk)
ISBN: 978-1-032-15158-8 (pbk)
ISBN: 978-1-003-24278-9 (ebk)

DOI: 10.1201/9781003242789

Typeset in Universe
by Apex CoVantage, LLC

Contents

Preface

This book sets echocardiography within a routine clinical context. It aims to synthesise guidelines into a pragmatic clinical approach to real patients, providing a step-by-step guide to performing, reporting, and interpreting a study. We wrote it imagining we were the calm voice of a senior echocardiographer teaching a junior. We also designed lists and tables as aides-memoires for the experienced echocardiographer or interpreting physician.

How We Handled Guidelines and Data

We took account of all up-to-date guidance from the ESC and ACC/AHA and also any other national or international body of authority that offered complementary or corroborative data or advice. Where guidelines disagreed or deviated from usual clinical practice, we conducted informal polls of internationally respected colleagues and reported the range of actual clinical practice marked by a logo to note the need for discussion within an individual department. If there were more recent normal ranges based on better collected data from larger populations than quoted in international guidelines, we used these. For example, we used the NORRE data for aortic diameters.

Expansion of Echocardiography

Since the third edition, echocardiography has expanded further into acute, intensive care, and emergency medicine. COVID-19 has necessitated limiting exposure of both patient and operator to infection and also caused a huge increase in waiting lists. This has sharpened the debate over the balance between abbreviated scans and comprehensive studies and highlighted the importance of collaboration between clinicians and echocardiographers. It is clear that the nature of the cardiac scan should be tailored to the clinical question, and this has led to the development of a range from basic, through focused, to standard and comprehensive echocardiograms. We discuss this in an expanded first chapter.

New Sections

We also include new sections on COVID-19, cardio-oncology, multivalve disease, and specialist valve clinics. We incorporated new international guidelines, grading criteria, and normal data. Since the third edition, there has been further development of cardiac CT and magnetic resonance, and we explain where these techniques are complementary to echocardiography and should be incorporated in a multimodality approach to normal clinical practice.

General Changes

The text has been reformatted to be more easily accessible, and numerous diagrams have been added or updated. Images and clips have been placed in a web-based archive.

This book will be relevant to all echocardiographers, including cardiac physiologists, clinical scientists, cardiologists, and clinicians in acute, critical care, general, and emergency medicine. It will also be useful to hospital and community physicians needing to interpret reports.

Acknowledgements

We should like to thank the people who took part in our online straw polls: Brian Campbell, Laura Dobson, Madalina Garbi, Jane Graham, Antoinette Kenny, Navroz Masani, Jim Newton, Petros Nihoyannopoulos, Keith Pearce, Bushra Rana, Dominik Schlosshan, Roxy Senior, Benoy Shah, and Rick Steeds. We are also grateful to colleagues who read through chapters and offered helpful advice: Claire Colebourne, Jane Draper, Yaso Emmanuel, Madalina Garbi, Jane Graham, Jeffrey Khoo, Simon MacDonald, Peter Saville, and David Sprigings. Any remaining mistakes are ours and not theirs. We should also like to thank Phillip Bentley, graphic designer, for updating the diagrams.

Authors

Camelia Demetrescu, BSc, MSc, HSSE, is Consultant Clinical Scientist in Cardiology, with specialist interest in echocardiography, at Guy's and St Thomas' Hospital. She has extensive NHS clinical, teaching, research, managerial, and leadership work experience across multiple London NHS tertiary trusts. She has a specialist interest in the management of patients with heart valve disease and interventional cardiology, inherited cardiomyopathies, heart transplant and assist devices, and most recently, in the research and development of AI technology. She is an active member of the European Association of Cardiovascular Imaging, the British Society of Echocardiography, British Heart Valve Society, Academy for Healthcare Science, and the National School of Healthcare Science.

Sandeep S Hothi, MA, PhD, FACC, FBSE, FESC, FRCP, is Consultant Cardiologist and Clinician-Scientist with expertise in advanced cardiac imaging. He studied at the University of Cambridge for undergraduate and postgraduate medical and scientific degrees: 1st Class BA (Hons) degree, clinical medical and surgical degrees (MB BChir) and a research degree (PhD) in cardiac cellular and whole heart physiology. He is a Consultant Cardiologist at New Cross Hospital, Wolverhampton, and Honorary Senior Clinical Lecturer at the University of Birmingham. He is accredited (SCMR, EACVI CMR, BSE, SCCT) in Echocardiography (transthoracic, transoesophageal, stress echo), Cardiac MRI and Cardiac CT. He holds societal roles with the British Society of Echocardiography as elected Trustee and Council Member, lead examiner for TOE accreditation, and Accreditation committee member.

John Chambers, MD, FRCP, FESC, is Emeritus Professor of Clinical Cardiology at Guy's and St Thomas' Hospital and KCL and was previously Head of Adult Echocardiography there. He helped in the foundation of the British Society of Echocardiography and was President from 2003 to 2005, responsible for establishing minimum standards for performing and reporting echocardiograms. He also helped set up individual transthoracic, transoesophageal, and departmental accreditation and a training system for basic echocardiography. He ran the London Echo Course for ten years and remains a faculty member of many national teaching courses. He has helped write a number of international documents on the imaging assessment of valve disease, including prosthetic valves. He was a founder-member and the first president of the British Heart Valve Society and helped set standards for specialist valve clinics and heart valve centres. He has written ten books on echocardiography, heart valve disease, and general medicine. He was awarded the British Cardiovascular Society 2023 Mackenzie medal for his career-long work in echocardiography and heart valve disease.

Disclaimer

The information in this book is based on a synthesis of data and guidelines available at the time of printing. The reader should be aware that clinical interpretation may change, and the writers cannot be held responsible for clinical events associated with the use of this book.

Icons and QR Codes

A number of new icons and QR codes have been used in this edition of the book to increase its usefulness to practitioners.

 Throughout the book, the **CHECKLIST** icon is used to signal checklist boxes summarising the main information on topics discussed.

 The **ALERT** icon flags up points to be particularly aware of or mistakes to avoid.

 The **THINK** icon marks a point of controversy or where consensus has not been reached.

 A point requiring discussion in an individual patient with integration into the clinical context is indicated by the **DISCUSSION** icon.

Abbreviations

AF	atrial fibrillation	LV	left ventricle/ventricular
Ao	aorta	LVDD	LV end-diastolic diameter
ARVC/D	arrhythmogenic right ventricular cardiomyopathy/dysplasia	LVEDV	LV end-diastolic volume
		LVEDVi	LV end-diastolic volume indexed to BSA
AR	aortic regurgitation	LVESV	LV end-systolic volume
AS	aortic stenosis	LVESVi	LV end-systolic volume indexed to BSA
ASD	atrial septal defect		
AVSD	atrioventricular septal defect	LVEDP	LV end-diastolic pressure
BSA	body surface area	LVOT	LV outflow tract
CABG	coronary artery bypass graft	LVSD	LV end-systolic diameter
CMR	cardiovascular magnetic resonance	MOA	mitral orifice area
		MR	mitral regurgitation
CSA	cross-sectional area	MS	mitral stenosis
CT	computerised tomography	PA	pulmonary artery
CW	continuous wave	PCI	percutaneous coronary intervention
DCM	dilated cardiomyopathy		
dP/dt	rate of developing pressure	PDA	persistent ductus arteriosus
ECG	electrocardiogram	PEEP	positive end-expiratory pressure
ECMO	extracorporeal membranous oxygenation		
		PET	positron emission tomography
EF	ejection fraction		
EOA	effective orifice area	PFO	patent fossa ovalis
EROA	effective regurgitant orifice area	PH	pulmonary hypertension
		PISA	proximal isovelocity surface area
FDG	fluorodeoxyglucose		
HCM	hypertrophic cardiomyopathy	PR	pulmonary regurgitation
IVC	inferior vena cava	PS	pulmonary stenosis
IVS	interventricular septum	RA	right atrium/atrial
LA	left atrium/left atrial	RF	regurgitant fraction
LAA	left atrial appendage	RV	right ventricle/ventricular
LBBB	left bundle branch block	RVOT	right ventricular outflow tract
LMS	left main stem		

RVEDV	RV end-diastolic volume		TS	tricuspid stenosis
RVESV	RV end-systolic volume		TTE	transthoracic echocardiogram/ echocardiography
RWT	relative wall thickness			
STJ	sinotubular junction		V_{max}	peak velocity
SV	stroke volume		VSD	ventricular septal defect
SVC	superior vena cava		VTI	velocity time integral
TAPSE	tricuspid annulus peak systolic excursion			(VTI_{aortic} measured on continuous wave Doppler through the aortic valve, VTI_{mitral} measured on continuous wave Doppler across the mitral valve, and $VTI_{subaortic}$ measured on pulsed Doppler in the LV outflow tract)
TAVI	transcatheter aortic valve implantation			
TDI	tissue Doppler imaging			
TOE	transoesophageal echocardiogram/ echocardiography			
TR	tricuspid regurgitation			

Defining the Study

Deciding the Level of Echocardiogram Required

- Cardiac ultrasound has now expanded in:
  - **Setting**—from the echocardiography laboratory to include cardiac and general wards; GP surgery and community echo clinics; the interventional laboratory, theatre, and intensive therapy unit; the emergency room and emergency settings, e.g. the road side or battlefield.
  - **Application**—from cardiology to acute, emergency, and intensive care medicine; to exclude significant structural disease in the community or the outpatient clinic.
  - **Hardware**—from high-end system through mid-range portable machines to handheld devices.
  - **Training**—from the use of cardiac ultrasound as an aid to resuscitation (by first responders) to basic studies (by the accredited physician in charge of the case or by accredited and highly experienced echocardiographers), to focused echocardiograms e.g. for community screening projects (often by nurses), to standard echocardiograms (by accredited echocardiographers), and to comprehensive studies (accredited and highly experienced echocardiographers).
- Cardiac ultrasound (e.g. FATE or FEEL protocols), usually including chest and abdominal imaging, is separate from echocardiography and part of emergency management.
- There are four levels of transthoracic echocardiography (TTE) (Table 1.1).
- Deciding the level of scan requires collaboration between clinician and echocardiographer (Figure 1.1) via:
  - A system of formal triage, including cases which do not need an echocardiogram at all (e.g. repeat studies with no clinical change).
  - Discussion about individual cases (e.g. in valve or heart failure specialist clinics).
- The decision on the level of scan will be based on:
  - The likelihood of disease. A basic TTE is sufficient to confirm the clinical impression of normality in low-risk cases, for example, flow murmurs or perceived palpitation in a young person[1, 2]. By comparison,

DOI: 10.1201/9781003242789-1

Table 1.1 **Aims of the four levels of echocardiogram (TTE) (Figure 1.1)**

Basic scan—can be performed with a handheld device with colour by an accredited* and highly experienced echocardiographer.**
- To detect pathology requiring immediate correction in the emergency setting (often performed by the physician in charge of the case).
- To determine what further investigations are indicated.
- To exclude the need for a minimum standard study in a patient at low clinical risk of disease.

Focused study—typically performed using a mid-range machine by an accredited echocardiographer* or operator specifically trained for a community screening project.
- To identify specific abnormalities in screening projects, for example, LV systolic and diastolic dysfunction, heart valve disease[3, 4].
- To detect change, for example, after an intervention in ITU, a new pericardial effusion after a cardiac intervention, an improvement in LV function after heart failure therapy, or in LV function on serial cardio-oncology scans.
- To detect significant change requiring a comprehensive study in patients with previous minimum standard studies, for example, moderate valve disease in a specialist valve clinic.

Minimum standard study—performed with at least a mid-range machine by an accredited echocardiographer,* if necessary, under supervision.
- This is the set of views and measurements (Tables 1.2 and 1.3) without which a study cannot be relied on to exclude significant pathology.

Comprehensive study—performed using a high-end machine by an accredited* and highly experienced echocardiographer.**
- This is a minimum standard study with additional disease-specific measurements (Table 1.4) as described in the chapters in this book.

* Accredited by a recognised national board or system, for example, the British Society of Echocardiography, European Association of Cardiovascular Imaging, American Society of Echocardiography, Australian BSc.

** Highly experienced echocardiographers are expected to notice mild abnormalities requiring a more extended study more readily than junior echocardiographers do.

a comprehensive study is more appropriate for a patient with a family history of cardiomyopathy.
- The results of previous studies. Confirming the stability of a previously noted abnormality does not usually need a comprehensive TTE.
- The clinical question. This might range from detecting signs of subtle disease (needing a comprehensive study) to whether the LV ejection fraction has changed (suitable for a focused study).
- Team working means that studies can be extended if unexpected pathology is detected.

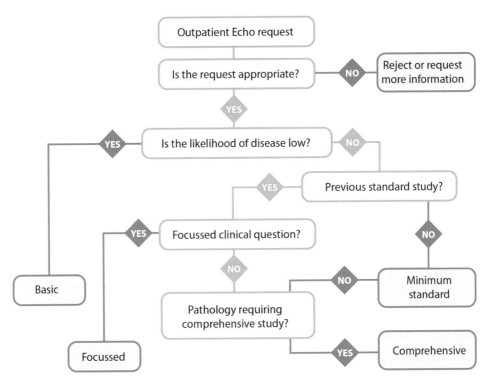

Figure 1.1 **Choosing the level of echocardiogram.**

The Basic Scan

- This is effectively an extension of the clinical examination and has these features[4-6]:
  - Basic views, usually: (1) parasternal long- and (2) short-axis (scanning from papillary muscles to aorta); (3) apical 4- then tilting to 5-chamber; (4) subcostal (Figure 1.2).
  - Systematic assessment of key cardiac structures: (1) LV size and function; (2) RV size and function and IVC; (3) valves; (4) presence of pericardial fluid.
  - Includes colour Doppler to detect significant valve disease.
- The result is classified as:
  - Major abnormality requiring immediate action, for example, pericardial tamponade, RV dilatation (as a surrogate for massive pulmonary embolism)[7].
  - Normal.
  - Requiring higher-level TTE (which can often be done immediately if equipment and operator appropriate), for example, more than trivial abnormalities, or basic scan apparently normal but patient unwell.

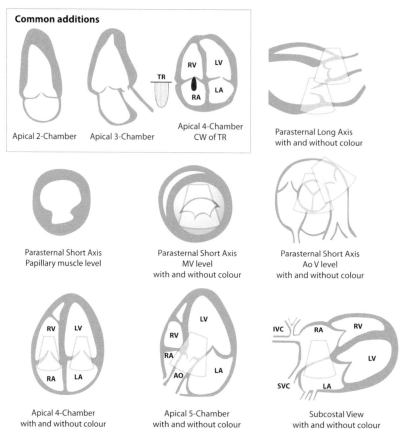

Common additions

Apical 2-Chamber   Apical 3-Chamber

RV   LV
TR
RA   LA

Apical 4-Chamber
CW of TR

Parasternal Long Axis
with and without colour

Parasternal Short Axis
Papillary muscle level

Parasternal Short Axis
MV level
with and without colour

Parasternal Short Axis
Ao V level
with and without colour

RV   LV
RA   LA

Apical 4-Chamber
with and without colour

LV
RV
RA
AO   LA

Apical 5-Chamber
with and without colour

IVC   RA   RV
LV
SVC   LA

Subcostal View
with and without colour

Figure 1.2 **A template showing views for the basic echocardiogram.**

- A suggested aide-memoire is given in Figure 1.2, but individual laboratories may add extra views or measurements as routine, for example, apical 2-chamber view or measurement of LV septal thickness or TR V_{max} if tricuspid regurgitation is detected or LA diameter in an electrophysiology request.

The Focused Study

- This always starts with a basic scan, to which specific 'add-ons' are determined by a clinical or research protocol or as directed by the clinician in charge of the case[8].
- Examples of 'add-ons' are:
  - TR V_{max} if more than mild TR shown[9].
  - RV tissue Doppler S' velocity, TAPSE, and TR V_{max} in sickle cell disease, in SLE, or in pulmonary embolism before and after thrombolysis.
  - Aortic dimensions and aortic regurgitation in a patient in an aortopathy clinic.

- LV measurements to estimate LV mass in hypertension[10].
- LV systolic function alone[9] or IVC reactivity[11] in follow-up heart failure clinics.

The Minimum Standard Study

- A minimum dataset of views and measurements is required to:
  - Confirm normal cardiac structure and function (Tables 1.2 and 1.3).
  - Reduce the risk of missing significant abnormalities.
  - Minimise inter- and intra-observer variability and enable accurate comparison of serial TTE.
  - Provide a structure for departmental quality audit.

- Clinically important measurements should be included in the text of the report.
  - Confining all measurements to a computer-generated section encourages their proliferation. Clinically important measurements may not be noticed especially if the requestor is a non-echocardiographer.
  - Each department should decide how many measurements to make and which should be brought into the text.
- Some protocols suggested by professional societies for a minimum standard study include measurements more properly classified as comprehensive.
- Each department needs to discuss how to manage measurements in atrial fibrillation.
  - Most aim to obtain measurements on cycles with instantaneous heart rates close to 60–70 bpm.
  - Once critical disease has been excluded by a basic TTE, it may be appropriate to bring the patient back once rate-controlled to continue the minimum standard study.

Table 1.2 **Minimum standard adult transthoracic echocardiogram (TTE) protocol**[12-15]

View	Essential imaging modalities**
P/S long axis	2D, colour Doppler
P/S RV inflow	2D, colour Doppler CW of TV if TR found
P/S RV outflow	2D, colour Doppler
P/S short axis at AV	2D, zoom, colour Doppler PW in RV outflow CW of PV and main PA CW of PR CW of TV if TR found

(Continued)

Table 1.2 Minimum standard adult transthoracic echocardiogram (TTE) protocol (Continued)

View	Essential imaging modalities**
P/S short axis at MV	2D, colour Doppler*
P/S short axis at pap muscles	2D, colour Doppler*
P/S short axis at apex	2D, colour Doppler*
Apical 4 chamber	2D, colour Doppler PW of MV CW of TV if TR found Doppler tissue MV and TV annulus
RV/RA modified Apical 4 chamber	2D, colour Doppler of TV M-mode TAPSE ± tissue Doppler CW of TV if TR found
Apical 5 chamber	2D, colour Doppler PW of LVOT CW of AV
Apical 2 chamber	2D, colour Doppler
Apical long axis	2D, colour Doppler
Subcostal long axis	2D, zoom on IVC and IAS, colour Doppler (IAS; hep vein) IVC reactivity by eye
Subcostal short axis	2D, colour Doppler
Subcostal abdominal aorta	2D, colour Doppler
Suprasternal notch–aortic arch	2D, colour Doppler

* To exclude a VSD.

** Extra views are suggested by some guidelines[12–15], e.g. CW of valves even if imaging and colour normal, LV strain.

Table 1.3 Minimum measurements for standard adult TTE protocol

Left ventricle
Diameters 2D: LVDD; LVSD; IVSd; PWd
2D volumes or 3D (when available) — BSA indexed*: LVEDVi and LVESVi
EF (using 2D or 3D volumes); $VTI_{subaortic}$
Mitral E/A and E/E' ratio using E' at septum ± lateral ± averaged according to local protocols

Left atrium
2D Volume (biplane method) or 3D — BSA indexed

Right ventricle
RV basal diameter; TAPSE and/or S' on tissue Doppler
TR V_{max}; acceleration time of PW in RV outflow tract
Inferior vena cava (inspiratory change): RA pressure assessment

Right atrium
2D area—2D Volume or 3D (when available)—BSA indexed

Aorta
2D diameter at sinuses, sinotubular junction, and ascending aorta indexed to height if at extremes of height

Aortic valve
CW V_{max}

* If BMI > 30 Kg/m², do not index to BSA, which underestimates the degree of cardiac remodelling.

The Comprehensive Study

● This is a minimum standard study plus extra views and measurements depending on the clinical question or known pathology (Table 1.4).

Table 1.4 **Views and measurements or descriptions as add-ons to the minimum standard according to the indication for the study**

Indication	Views	Measurements/ observation
Possible LV dysfunction (indication heart failure, cardiomyopathy)	● Zoom LVOT and MV in HCM ● Zoom LV apex +/– colour Doppler in cardiomyopathy or myocardial infarction ● Modified LV views in suspected post-infarct VSD ● Contrast study for endocardial border delineation/thrombus	● RWT and LV mass BSA indexed (g/m²) ● 2D/3D dyssynchrony parameters ● 3D volume and ejection fraction ● GLS ● LVOT obstruction at rest/Valsalva in HCM
Possible RV dysfunction	● RV-specific views (page 35) ● Zoom RV apex ● M-mode of annulus in zoomed 4-chamber view	● RV 2D P/S long- and short-axis diameters ● RV fractional area change ● RV EF on 3D
Aortic stenosis	● Zoom in LVOT ● CW at apex and RICS	● LVOT diameter ● V_{max}, mean ΔP, EOA ● CW to exclude coarctation ● Evidence of PHT

(Continued)

Table 1.4 **Views and measurements or descriptions as add-ons to the minimum standard according to the indication for the study** (Continued)

Indication	Views	Measurements/observation
Aortic regurgitation	• Zoom aortic root and ascending aorta • AR CW • Colour M-mode suprasternal	• Colour jet width • AR pressure half-time • Flow reversal in descending aorta (PW and colour)
Mitral regurgitation	• Zoom MV in all views • PW in pulmonary vein	• Detailed valve morphology and mechanism of MR • MV annulus size • Tenting height/area • PISA/vena contracta • Evidence of PHT
Mitral stenosis	• Zoom MV in all views	• MV orifice planimetered area • V_{max}, pressure 1/2 time (and estimated area), mean gradient • Evidence of PHT
Pericardial constriction	• PW at MV (slow sweep speed) • PW in hepatic veins • MV annulus tissue Dopplor	• Look for septal bounce • Resp variability in transmitral PW • Soptal and latoral tissue Doppler E'

Organisation of a Report

1. **The minimum standard report[16] should include:**
   - **Basic data:**
     - Patient name, date of birth, and hospital number.
     - Echocardiographer ID (initials/name).
     - Information regarding echocardiographic machine, type of image storage media, and location is recommended to facilitate review.
   - **Minimum patient observations:**
     - Age and sex and body dimensions (height, weight, body surface area).
     - A good-quality ECG trace for heart rate and rhythm.

- **Indication.** A TTE should not usually be performed without a written request (except in life-threatening emergencies). The request should include:
  - The indication (ideally including previous medical history).
  - Clinical questions to be answered.
  - Referrer details (name, title, address, email).
- **Minimum measurements** (see Table 1.3). Clinically important measurements need to be given in the text of the report, and it is not sufficient to have these in a list of machine-generated numbers.
- **The main text** should include:
  - A description of image quality (poor, adequate, good).
  - A description of the morphological and functional findings of all parts of the heart and great vessels.
  - If it was not possible to image a region, this should be stated.
  - Preliminary interpretation can be included where it aids understanding, for example, 'rheumatic mitral valve'. The grade of stenosis or regurgitation can also be stated as long as the observations used are included.
  - No consensus exists about reporting minor abnormalities (e.g. mild mitral annulus calcification), normal variants (e.g. Chiari network), or normal findings (e.g. trivial mitral regurgitation). We suggest describing these in the text but omitting them from the conclusion.
- **The summary:**
  - **Must answer the clinical question** posed by the referrer.
  - **Must emphasise abnormal findings** in descending order of clinical importance.
  - Should **identify the abnormality** (e.g. mitral regurgitation), **its cause** (e.g. mitral prolapse), and the **secondary effects** (e.g. LV dilatation and hyperactivity).
  - Should compare with previous findings if available.
  - Should avoid abbreviations and be understood by non-specialist healthcare professionals.
  - Should not usually include clinical advice. This requires the echocardiographic findings to be integrated with the broader clinical assessment, which is not available to the echocardiographer. However, it may be reasonable to offer implicit **management advice** in the report, for example: 1) 'Valve suitable for balloon valvotomy based on echocardiographic assessment.'; 2) 'Valve suitable for repair based on echocardiographic assessment.'; 3) 'Severe mitral regurgitation with LV dilatation at thresholds suitable for surgery.'

Escalation for Urgent Clinical Advice

- Each laboratory should have a system of identifying **critical findings** (Table 1.5) and communicating them to the referrer or a cardiologist.
- Documentation of communication of the critical findings **must be recorded in the report and/or in the patient's medical record**.

Table 1.5 Examples of critical findings requiring urgent clinical advice

Critically unwell patient, regardless of echocardiographic findings
Pericardial effusion: large or with evidence of tamponade
Aortic dissection or grossly dilated ascending aorta or abscess
Previously undiagnosed severely impaired LV systolic function
Serious complications of an acute coronary syndrome: • Ventricular septal rupture • Papillary muscle rupture • False aneurysm
RV dilatation or hypokinesis in a patient with suspected pulmonary embolism
New severe valve disease
New cardiac mass or thrombus

Understanding the Report for Non-Echocardiographers

1. **Some findings are almost never of clinical importance:**
   - Mild tricuspid and pulmonary regurgitation, which are both normal findings. Isolated moderate tricuspid regurgitation is also within normal limits if the RV is not dilated and the left heart is normal.
   - Mild mitral regurgitation with a normal valve appearance and normal LV size and function.
   - 'Sigmoid septum' (or 'septal bulge'), which is common in the elderly and may cause a murmur.
   - Trivial pericardial fluid especially localised around the right atrium (in the absence of chest pain, suggesting pericarditis).
   - An incidental patent foramen ovale in the absence of a relevant clinical history (TIA or stroke, peripheral embolism, diving).

2. **What do class 1, 2, and 3 diastolic dysfunction mean?**
   - Echocardiographers are now encouraged to describe the pattern of LV filling using a system of classification. 'Slow filling', which is common and arguably normal in the elderly, has become 'class 1 diastolic dysfunction'.
   - Class 2 and 3 dysfunctions suggest high LV filling pressures, but these classes are easily confused with diastolic heart failure, which is a clinical diagnosis that cannot be made on TTE alone.
   - If the patient is well, it is likely that LV diastolic dysfunction is an incidental observation of no clinical significance.

3. **How do I interpret a probability of pulmonary hypertension?**
   - If the request was to detect pulmonary hypertension (e.g. in the context of SLE), then the recommendation is to report a low, intermediate, or high probability of pulmonary hypertension (see Chapter 5). TTE cannot estimate PA pressure reliably enough to make a management-changing diagnosis. Further investigation potentially with a right heart catheter is then needed.
   - If the patient has valve disease:
     - In mitral stenosis, a PA systolic pressure >50 mmHg at rest is an indication for balloon valvotomy even in the absence of symptoms.
     - In severe aortic stenosis (AS), a PA systolic pressure >60 mmHg indicates a high risk of dying, unless surgery or a TAVI is performed.
     - A rise in TR V_{max} is a secondary sign of deterioration in any type of valve disease.
   - If the request was for any other reason and no other cardiac abnormalities are reported, seek a cardiac opinion.

4. **In specific diseases, there are echocardiographic findings that might trigger changes in management** (Table 1.6).

Table 1.6 **Alerts in the echo report by pathology**

Asymptomatic severe valve disease. Check that LV size and function are normal
In severe mitral regurgitation, surgery may be indicated for a systolic diameter >40 mm or LV ejection fraction approaching 60% (see Chapter 9).
In severe aortic regurgitation, surgery may be indicated for a systolic diameter >50 mm, diastolic diameter >65 mm, or LV ejection fraction approaching 50% (see Chapter 8).
Moderate disease may still be significant if the LV size and function are abnormal.

(Continued)

Table 1.6 Alerts in the echo report by pathology (Continued)

In suspected heart failure:
Diastolic heart failure cannot usually be diagnosed on the TTE alone without clinical features and BNP levels. Diastolic dysfunction does not necessarily imply diastolic heart failure.
Heart rate and rhythm may interfere with the assessment of ventricular systolic and diastolic function.
The LV ejection fraction depends on preload and afterload, both of which can change quickly according to a patient's clinical condition.
Estimations of LV ejection fraction are highly operator-dependent, and small changes should not be over-interpreted.

Patient's fitness for surgery:
The TTE evaluates only some aspects of the cardiovascular system. It cannot detect myocardial ischaemia.

Is there a cardiac source for embolism?
TTE is the modality of choice to demonstrate intraventricular mass or thrombus when images are satisfactory.
TTE does not image the left atrial appendage adequately. TOE may be required if it changes clinical management.
When patent foramen ovale must be excluded as a source of cryptogenic stroke in young patients, transthoracic bubble contrast study is recommended (see pages 56, 57).

In suspected pericarditis or pericardial effusion:
Uncomplicated pericarditis has no pathognomonic features on TTE.
TTE can detect complications of pericarditis, such as a pericardial effusion.
Tamponade is a clinical diagnosis, though TTE is useful to assess haemodynamic changes.

References

1. Draper J, Subbiah S, Bailey R & Chambers J. The murmur clinic. Validation of a new model for detecting heart valve disease. Heart 2019;105(1):56–9.
2. Smith J, Subbiah S, Hayes A, Campbell B & Chambers J. Feasibility of an outpatient point-of-care echocardiography service. J Am Soc Echo 2019;32(7):909–10.
3. Ploutz M, Ju JC, Scheel J, et al. Handheld echocardiographic screening for rheumatic heart disease by non-experts. Heart 2016;102(1):35–9.
4. Hammadah M, Ponce C, Sorajja P, et al. Point-of-care ultrasound: Closing guideline gaps in screening for valvular heart disease. Clin Cardiol 2020;43(12):1368–75.

5. Spencer KT, Kimura BJ, Korcarz CE, et al. Focused cardiac ultrasound: Recommendations from the American Society of Echocardiography J Am Soc Echo 2013;26(6):567–81.
6. Cardim N, Dalen H, Voigt J-U, et al. The use of handheld devices: A position statement of the European Association of Cardiovascular Imaging (2018 update). Europ Heart J 2019;20(3):245–52.
7. Hall DP, Jordan H, Alam S & Gillies MA. The impact of focused echocardiography using the focused intensive care echo protocol on the management of critically ill patients, and comparison with full echocardiographic studies by BSE-accredited sonographers. J Intensive Care Soc 2017;18(3):206–11.
8. Rice JA, Brewer J, Speaks T, et al. The POCUS consult: How point of care ultrasound helps guide medical decision making. Int J Gen Med 2021;14:9789–806.
9. Dowling K, Colling A, Walters H, et al. Piloting structural focused TTE in outpatients during the COVID-19 pandemic: Old habits die hard. Br J Cardiol 2021;28:148–52.
10. Senior R, Galasko G, Hickman M, et al. Community screening for left ventricular hypertrophy in patients with hypertension using hand-held echocardiography. J Am Soc Echo 2004;17(1):56–61.
11. Gundersen GH, Norekval TM, Haug HH, et al. Adding point of care ultrasound to assess volume status in heart failure patients in a nurse-led outpatient clinic. A randomised study. Heart 2016;102(1):29–34.
12. Harkness A, Ring L, Augustine D, Oxborough D, Robinson S, Sharma V & Stout M. Normal reference intervals for cardiac dimensions and function for use in echocardiographic practice: A guideline from the British Society of Echocardiography. Echo Research and Practice 2020;7(1):G1–18.
13. Robinson S., Bushra R., Oxborough D, et al. Guidelines and recommendations. A practical guideline for performing a comprehensive transthoracic echocardiogram in adults: The British Society of Echocardiography minimum dataset. Echo Research and Practice 2020;7(4):G59–93.
14. Lang RM, Badano LP, Mor-Avi V, et al. Recommendations for cardiac chamber quantification by echocardiography in adults: An update from the American Society of Echocardiography and the European Association of Cardiovascular Imaging. Eur Heart J CVI 2015;16(3):233–70.
15. Mitchell C, Rahko PS, Blanwet LA, et al. Guidelines for performing a comprehensive transthoracic echocardiographic examination in adults: Recommendations from the American Society of Echocardiography. J Am Soc Echo 2019;32(1):P1–764.
16. Galderisi M, Cosyns B, Edvardsen T, et al. Standardization of adult transthoracic echocardiography reporting in agreement with recent chamber quantification, diastolic function, and heart valve disease recommendations: An expert consensus document of the European Association of Cardiovascular Imaging. Europ Heart J CVI 2017;18(12):1301–10.

Left Ventricular Dimensions and Function

2

The assessment includes:

- **LV linear cavity dimensions**
- **LV wall thickness**
- **LV volumes**—2D biplane Simpson's or 3D full volume, when available
- **LV function**—systolic and diastolic

LV Linear Cavity Dimensions

- Measure at the base of the heart using 2D-guided measurements (Figure 2.1).
- In patients with a sigmoid septum, measurements should be performed slightly towards the apex, just beyond the septal bulge[1].

- Commonly used normal ranges and grades of abnormality suggested by ASE/EACVI are given in Table 2.1. Grades are useful for communication with clinicians despite not necessarily correlating closely with outcomes. **Whether to use grades or a simpler classification as normal, dilated, or severely dilated needs to be discussed by individual labs.**

- The ASE/EACVI data are used in current ESC guidelines on diagnosis and management, for example, in valve disease and cardiomyopathies.
- However, the BSE 2020 guidelines, derived from the NORRE dataset, give larger end-systolic dimensions than in Table 2.1, for example, severely dilated LVSD >46 mm in women, and >50 mm in men[3]. Individual labs need to agree whether to use ASE/EACVI or NORRE ranges.
- ASE/EACVI recommend that chamber measurements should be indexed to BSA (most commonly using the Dubois–Dubois formula)[5]. This is not done routinely in clinical practice because:
    - In mitral and aortic valve disease, outcomes and the timing of interventions are related to absolute LV dimensions[4].
    - For a BMI >30 kg/m^2, indexing may overcorrect an abnormally large dimension.
    - However, indexing should be done to help identify borderline abnormalities in patients, particularly at extremes of size (e.g. DCM family screening).

DOI: 10.1201/9781003242789-2

15

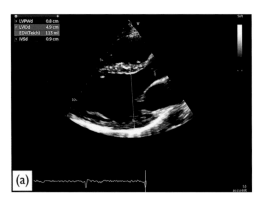
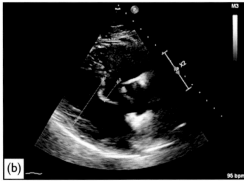

Figure 2.1 Sites for making 2D measurements. (a) Linear internal measurements of the LV should be acquired in the parasternal long-axis view perpendicular to the LV long axis and measured at the level of the mitral valve leaflet tips. (b) In patients with sigmoid septum, LV cavity measurements should be performed slightly towards the apex, just beyond the septal bulge. Guidelines suggest measuring from inner to inner edge. Diastolic measurements are timed with the onset of the QRS complex, and systolic measurements with the end of the T wave on the electrocardiogram.

Table 2.1 Grading of LV cavity diameters suggested by ASE/EACVI[2]

	Normal	Mildly dilated	Moderately dilated	Severely dilated
Women				
LVDD (mm)	38–52	53–56	57–61	>61
LVSD (mm)	22–35	36–38	39–41	>41
Men				
LVDD (mm)	42–58	59–63	64–68	>68
LVSD (mm)	25–40	41–43	44–45	>45

Abbreviations: LVDD, left ventricle end-diastolic diameter; LVSD, left ventricle end-systolic diameter.

LV Wall Thickness

- Measurements should be taken at the base of the heart.
- A guide to grading thickness is given in Table 2.2.
- Patterns of hypertrophy are given in Table 2.3 and Figure 2.2.
- If the LV looks hypertrophied but the measured thickness is normal, this is usually because of concentric remodelling. This is a precursor to hypertrophy in pressure overload. It is defined by a relative wall thickness (RWT) >0.45.

Table 2.2 **Grading LV wall thickness suggested by ASE/EACVI[1, 2]**

Normal	Mildly thickened	Moderately thickened	Severely thickened
Women			
6–9 mm	10–12 mm	13–15 mm	≥16 mm
Men			
6–10 mm	11–13 mm	14–16 mm	≥17 mm

Table 2.3 **Patterns of hypertrophy**

Symmetrical	
Concentric	Thick wall and reduced LV cavity size in response to pressure load (e.g. aortic stenosis, systemic hypertension). Defined by relative wall thickness >0.45.
Eccentric	Occurs to offset the high-wall stress resulting from LV dilatation (e.g. in volume load in aortic or mitral regurgitation). Relative wall thickness <0.45. Wall stress = LV pressure × (LVDD/wall thickness).
Asymmetrical	Localised (e.g. LV apex or septum).

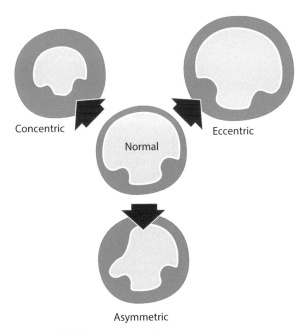

Figure 2.2 **Patterns of LV hypertrophy.**

Table 2.4 **Grading LV mass suggested by ASE/EACVI using linear dimensions*[2]**

	Normal	Mild hypertrophy	Moderate hypertrophy	Severe hypertrophy
Women				
LV mass (g)	67–162	163–186	187–210	>210
LV mass/ BSA (g/m²)	43–95	96–108	109–121	>121
Men				
LV mass (g)	88–224	225–258	259–292	>292
LV mass/ BSA (g/m²)	49–115	116–131	132–148	>148

* LV mass = $0.83 \times [(LVDD + IVS + PW)^3 - LVDD^3]$.

- RWT = (2 × posterior wall thickness)/LV diastolic diameter.
- Calculation of LV mass is not routinely necessary in clinical practice.
- A guide to grading LV mass is given in Table 2.4.

LV hypertrophy in obese patients (BMI >30 kg/m²) is a pathological process and may be underestimated by indexing to BSA. Instead, LV mass should be indexed to height with LV hypertrophy defined by LV mass >50 g/m in men and >47 g/m in women[6].

LV Volumes

- If the linear dimensions are abnormal or there is relevant pathology (e.g. cardiomyopathy or valve disease), LV volume should be measured either by 2D or 3D and indexed to BSA.
- When ≥2 contiguous endocardial segments cannot be visualised in the apical views, 3D calculations are not feasible and contrast agents should be considered for 2D Simpson's method if an accurate result is needed[1].

- The BSE 2020 guideline, based on the NORRE dataset, gives a normal range for LVEDVi of 30–79 mL/m² for men and 29–70 mL/m² for women[3]. The cut point for severe dilatation is >91 mL/m² for women and 103 mL/m² for men[3].

- Individual labs need to agree whether to report individual ASE/EACVI grades (Table 2.5) or NORRE normal, abnormal, and severely dilated.
- International guidelines for cardiomyopathy still use ESC data.

Table 2.5 **ASE/EACVI grades for LV 2D-derived cavity volume**[2]

	Normal	Mildly dilated	Moderately dilated	Severely dilated
Women				
LVEDVi (mL/m²)	29–61	62–70	71–80	>80
LVESVi (mL/m²)	8–24	25–32	33–40	>40
LVEDV (mL)	46–106	–	–	>130
LVESV (mL)	14–42	–	–	>67
Men				
LVEDVi (mL/m²)	34–74	75–89	90–100	>100
LVESVi (mL/m²)	11–31	32–38	39–45	>45
LVEDV (mL)	62–150	–	–	>200
LVESV (mL)	21–61	–	–	>85

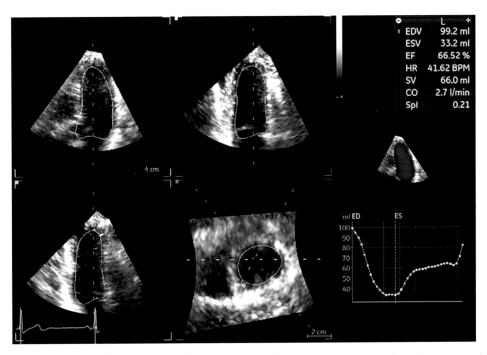

Figure 2.3 **LV 3D volume.** 3D image acquisition focuses on including the entire left ventricle within the pyramidal dataset. Volumetric measurements are based on tracings of the interface between the compacted myocardium and the LV cavity. Use gated acquisition full volume over two to six cardiac cycles.

- Normal ranges for 3D volumes vary widely but are larger than 2D volumes. Suggested upper limits of normal for LVEDVi are 79 mL/m^2 for men and 71 mL/m^2 for women, and for LVESVi are 32 mL/m^2 for men and 28 mL/m^2 for women[2].
- Serial comparison of 3D LV volumes and EF is useful in highly specialist clinics (e.g. cardio-oncology, inherited cardiac conditions, valve clinics). Measurements should be performed only when the 3D dataset is of good quality, using the same equipment, ideally by the same operator, and analysed on the same software.

LV Systolic Function

1. Regional LV wall motion

- Look at each arterial territory in every view.
- Describe wall motion abnormalities by segment (Figure 2.4) according to their systolic thickening and phase (Table 2.6).
- Some centres assign a score to these descriptive categories. The most common system is given in Table 2.6.

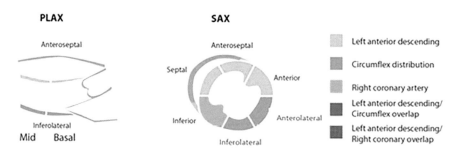

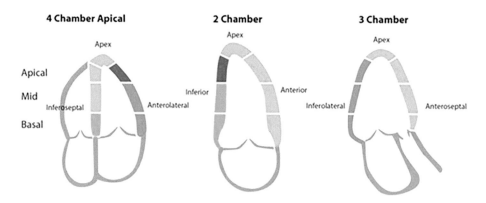

Figure 2.4 **Arterial territories of the heart.** The nomenclature of the 17-segment model is now established. Sometimes the apex is unreported if it is not seen well. However, small apical aneurysms or apical thrombus may occur, and a stress test may only be positive at the apex. The usual arterial territories are superimposed.

Table 2.6 **A commonly used wall motion scoring system**

Wall motion	Score
Normal	1
Hypokinesis (<50% normal movement)	2
Akinesis (absent movement)	3
Dyskinesis (movement out of phase with the rest of the ventricle)	4
Aneurysmal (paradoxical motion)	5

Table 2.7 **Grading LV ejection fraction—biplane Simpson's method[3]**

Normal	Borderline*	Impaired	Severely impaired**
≥55%	50–54%	36–49%	≤35%

* The values need to be interpreted with caution in individual cases. An EF 50–54% may be normal in an athletic young subject, but may be abnormal if previously recorded as 60% without changes in loading conditions or pre-chemotherapy.

** The cut point for severe impairment is either 30% or 35%, according to the published guideline[2, 3]. Therapeutic decisions, for example, implantation of an AICD or CRT, usually use 35% as the cut point. If EF is obtained using 3D imaging, these should be compared to vendor-specific reference intervals.

2. Global LV systolic function

The minimum standard measurements are:

- **LV ejection fraction** (Table 2.7 for a guide to grading). LV systolic function may still be impaired despite a normal LV ejection fraction if there are:
    - Wall motion abnormalities
    - Low VTI$_{subaortic}$
    - Subtle abnormalities, for example, on Doppler tissue or GLS (see page 22)

- **Pulsed tissue Doppler systolic velocity** (S'). Guidelines recommend averaging the values at the lateral and septal mitral valve annulus in the apical 4-chamber view. Some centres report just the septal value in the text of the report. Methods of measurement and limitations are given in Figure 2.5. Normal values are given in Table 2.8.

- **Velocity time integral or stroke distance** (VTI$_{subaortic}$). Measured using pulsed Doppler in the LVOT outflow tract in the 5-chamber view.
    - Stroke volume can be calculated using the LVOT radius (r):
        - Stroke volume = $\pi r^2 \times$ VTI$_{subaortic}$
        - Cardiac output is stroke volume × heart rate

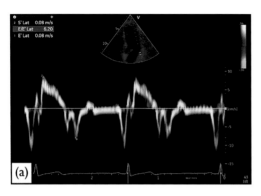
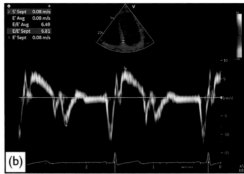

Figure 2.5 **TDI S' and E'.** Peak systolic velocity of mitral annulus by pulsed TDI (cm/s) is obtained by aligning the cursor to the direction of movement of the LV wall and placing the sample volume at or within 10 mm of the insertion site of the mitral valve leaflets. Optimise the velocity scale and baseline to demonstrate the full signal. Measurements are obtained at end-expiration. Limitations: The S', E' velocities or E/E' ratio should not usually be measured in the presence of marked mitral annular calcification, prosthetic mitral valves, annuloplasty rings, and severe mitral valve disease. The lateral site should not be used in pericardial constriction; the septal site should be avoided in paced hearts. The site adjacent to the myocardial wall infarction should not be used.

Table 2.8 **Normal LV TDI average (lateral and septal) systolic velocity according to age[3]**

Parameter	20–40 years	40–60 years	>60 years
S' (cm/s)	≥6.4	≥5.7	≥4.9

- A normal VTI$_{subaortic}$ is[7]:
  - 17–23 cm with normal heart rate, 55–95 bpm.
  - >18 cm with heart rate <55 bpm.
  - <22 cm with heart rate >95 bpm to ensure a normal SV and CO.
- In acute decompensated heart failure or acute pulmonary embolism, a VTI$_{subaortic}$ <15 cm is associated with a poor prognosis[7].

Other measures are used to detect subtle LV dysfunction in the presence of normal or borderline LV ejection fraction:

- **Global longitudinal strain (GLS)** is used in cardio-oncology and selected groups of patients with inherited cardiac conditions when comparison with previous studies can be made using the same system and analysed using the same software.
  - Cut-off values from cardio-oncology guidelines are given in Table 2.9. There are no agreed normal ranges for other clinical situations[1–3].

- **Left ventricular dP/dt** is a relatively load-independent measure of the development of LV pressure (Figure 2.6) and is used in LV disease and valve disease.

- Normal is >1,200 mmHg/s, equivalent to a 25 ms delay between 1.0 and 3.0 m/s (Table 2.10).

Table 2.9 Cut-offs for adult GLS cardio-oncology clinics[8]

Normal GLS	Borderline GLS	Abnormal GLS
GLS <−18%	−16% to −18%	GLS >−16%

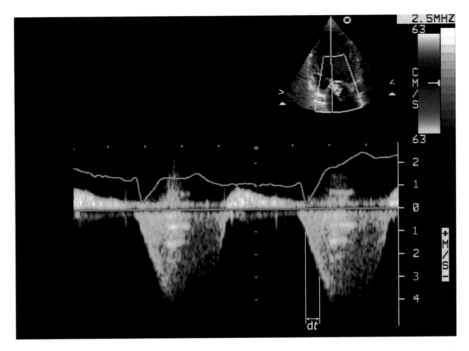

Figure 2.6 **Estimating LV dP/dt.** Measure the time (dt) between 1.0 m/s and 3.0 m/s on the upstroke, which represents a pressure change of 32 mmHg [$(4 \times 3.0^2) - (4 \times 1.0^2)$] using the short form of the modified Bernoulli theorem. dP/dt is then 32/dt.

Table 2.10 Guide to grading LV function by mitral regurgitant signal

	Normal	Abnormal	Severely abnormal
dP/dt (mmHg/s)	>1,200	800–1,200	<800
Time from 1 to 3 m/s (ms)	<25	25–40	>40

LV Diastolic Function

- The minimum standard study includes:
  - Transmitral E and A peak velocity, E deceleration time, and E/A ratio.

- Peak E' on the TDI signal at the level of the mitral valve annulus.
- LA volume using biplane method (apical 4-chamber and 2-chamber views) indexed to BSA (see Chapter 6). Normal is <34 mL/m². Dilatation occurs in diastolic LV dysfunction.
- TR V$_{max}$ and estimated pulmonary pressure (see pages 43–45).

- Use these measures to describe the filling pattern as normal, slow-filling, or restrictive (Table 2.11) and state if there is evidence of raised LV filling pressures. Some labs grade LV diastolic dysfunction, but this carries the risk of equating this with diastolic heart failure.
- In atrial fibrillation, diastole is already abnormal. It is still worth measuring E, E deceleration, and E' to look for restrictive filling.
- If the LV ejection fraction is <50%, the diagnosis of heart failure is already made, but restrictive filling defines a group with a high risk of decompensation or death.

Table 2.11 **Definitions of filling patterns**

LV filling pattern	MV E/A ratio	MV E (cm/s)	E/E' ratio	LV filling pressure
Normal	>0.8	>50	<10	Normal
Slow filling (grade I)	≤0.8	≤50	<10	Normal
Pseudonormal (grade II)	>0.8 but <2	>50	>14*	Raised
Restrictive (grade III)	E/A ≥2	>50	>14	Raised

* If E/E' is between 10 and 14, use additional cut points: TR V$_{max}$ >2.8 m/s; LA vol indexed >34 mL/m²; TDI E' sep <7 cm/s or E' lat <10 cm/s. The more of these are abnormal, the more likely there is to be diastolic dysfunction[9].

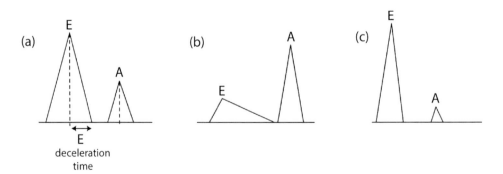

Figure 2.7 **Left ventricular filling patterns.** (a) Normal; (b) slow filling (low peak E velocity, long deceleration time, high peak A velocity); (c) restrictive (high peak E velocity with short E deceleration time with low or absent A wave).

- Restrictive filling is sometimes subdivided into reversible (normalises with a fall in preload, for example, after a Valsalva manoeuvre) and irreversible. Irreversible restrictive filling is associated with a particularly high risk of events.

LVEF >50%: Diastolic Heart Failure (HFpEF)?

This is a clinical diagnosis which uses the TTE[10] but cannot be made with the TTE alone.

- The non-echocardiographic factors used are:
  - Symptoms and clinical signs of heart failure
  - Cardiovascular risk factors: body mass index >30 Kg/m^2, hypertension, atrial fibrillation
  - Absence of other causes of breathlessness, including valve disease
  - Raised level of B-type natriuretic peptide
  - Other tests, including CMR, if amyloid is suspected; right heart catheter with exercise to detect a rise in pulmonary capillary wedge pressure

- Suggestive TTE features include concentric LV remodelling or hypertrophy and LA dilatation.
- TTE measurements suggesting diastolic dysfunction are given in Table 2.12.
- If LV diastolic function is indeterminate, assess pulmonary vein flow (Figure 2.8):
  - The peak velocity of the pulmonary vein atrial flow reversal
  - The duration of atrial flow reversal (PV Ar duration)
  - The duration of the transmitral A wave (transmitral duration)
  - The most reliable measure of diastolic dysfunction (Table 2.12) is the pulmonary venous Ar reversal duration–transmitral A duration (Ar–A) >30 ms.

Table 2.12 **Diastolic function using transmitral and pulmonary vein pulsed Doppler[11]**

	Transmitral and TDI pattern	Ar–A duration	PV Ar peak velocity
Normal	Normal	Normal	<0.35 m/s
Mild dysfunction	Slow filling	Normal	<0.35 m/s
Moderate dysfunction	Pseudo-normal	Prolonged >30 ms	>0.35 m/s
Severe dysfunction	Restrictive	Prolonged >30 ms	>0.35 m/s

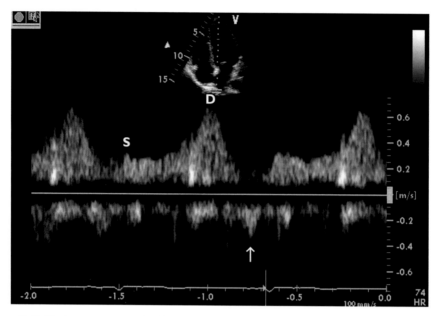

Figure 2.8 **Pulmonary vein flow patterns.** The systolic (S) and diastolic (D) peaks of forward flow are marked. Atrial reversal (arrow) has a peak velocity of 0.35 m/s.

MISTAKES TO AVOID

- Incorporating a false LV tendon or RV trabeculation in the septal measurement.
- Cutting the septum or LV cavity obliquely.
- Measuring the LV internal dimensions at the level of a sigmoid septum.
- Diagnosing diastolic heart failure from the echocardiographic filling pattern alone.
- In a patient with clinical heart failure and preserved LV ejection fraction, forgetting to consider pericardial constriction. Check for a dilated IVC and septal bounce (Chapter 17).
- Diagnosing systolic dysfunction from a borderline LV ejection fraction in an athletic subject (see page 63).

CHECKLIST FOR REPORTING LV FUNCTION

1. LV and LA dimensions.
2. Global and regional LV systolic function.
3. LV diastolic function +/− high filling pressure.
4. RV function and PA pressure.

References

1. Mitchell C, Rahko PS, Blauwet LA, et al. Guidelines for performing a comprehensive transthoracic echocardiographic examination in adults: Recommendations from the American Society of Echocardiography. J Am Soc Echo 2019;32(1):1–64.
2. Lang R, Badano L, Mor-Avi V, et al. Recommendations for cardiac chamber quantification by echocardiography in adults: An update from the American Society of Echocardiography and the European Association of Cardiovascular Imaging. Europ Heart J CVI 2015;16(3):233–71.
3. Harkness A, Ring L, Augustine DX, et al. Guidelines and recommendations: Normal reference intervals for cardiac dimensions and function for use in echocardiographic practice: A guideline from the British Society of Echocardiography. Echo Research and Practice 2020;7(1):G1–18.
4. Nishimura RA, Otto CM, Bonow RO, et al. AHA/ACC focused update of the 2014 ACC/ AHA guideline for the management of patients with valvular heart disease: A report of the American College of Cardiology/American Heart Association Task Force on Clinical Practice Guidelines. Circulation 2017;135(25):e1159–95.
5. Ristow B, Ali S, Na B, Turakhia MP, Whooley MA & Schiller NB. Predicting heart failure hospitalization and mortality by quantitative echocardiography: Is body surface area the indexing method of choice? The heart and soul study. J Am Soc Echocardiography 2010;23(4):406–13.
6. Singh M, Sethi A, Mishra AK, et al. Echocardiographic imaging challenges in obesity: Guideline recommendations and limitations of adjusting to body size. J Am Heart Assoc 2020;9(2):1–9.
7. Blanco P. Rationale for using the velocity–time integral and the minute distance for assessing the stroke volume and cardiac output in point-of-care settings. Ultrasound Journal 2020;12(1):21.
8. Liu J, Barac A, Thavendiranathan P & Scherrer-Crosbie M. Strain imaging in cardio-oncology. J Am Coll Cardiol Cardio-oncology 2020;2(5):677–89.
9. Nagueh SF, Smiseth AO, Appleton CP, et al. ASE/EACVI guidelines and standards: Recommendations for the evaluation of left ventricular diastolic function by echocardiography: An update from the American Society of Echocardiography and the European Association of Cardiovascular Imaging. J Am Soc Echo 2016;29(4):277–314.
10. Pieske B, Tschope C, de Boer RA, et al. How to diagnose heart failure with preserved ejection fraction: The HFA–PEFF diagnostic algorithm: A consensus recommendation from the Heart Failure Association (HFA) of the European Society of Cardiology (ESC). Europ Heart J 2019;40(40):3297–317.
11. Redfield MM, Jacobsen SJ, Burnett JC, Mahoney DW, Bailey KR & Rodeheffer RJ. Burden of systolic and diastolic ventricular dysfunction in the community: Appreciating the scope of the heart failure epidemic. J Am Med Assoc 2003;289(2):194–202.

Acute Coronary Syndrome

3

Echocardiography is indicated:

- To help determine whether a mildly raised troponin level is caused by a new cardiac event or non-cardiac illness.
- After myocardial infarction to determine residual LV function and to look for complications.
- In acute chest pain with suspected myocardial infarction (with non-diagnostic ECG or ST segment changes), and when the scan can be performed during pain, to aid the differentiation between myocardial ischaemia and other causes (e.g. pericarditis or aortic dissection).
- As an emergency in cardiac decompensation, to look for acute complications, for example, papillary muscle rupture or ventricular septal or free wall rupture[1].

1. Assess regional LV systolic function

The working diagnosis is confirmed by a regional wall motion abnormality, without scarring, in an arterial territory:

- Describe the segments affected (see Figure 2.4, page 20).
- Comment on the other regions. Compensatory hyperkinesis is a good prognostic sign. Hypokinesis of a territory other than of the acute ischaemia could suggest multivessel disease and is a poor prognostic sign.
- Are there thin segments implying previous coronary events?
- Consider enhancement with transpulmonary contrast if two or more adjacent segments are not well seen or LV thrombus is suspected.
- A wall motion abnormality affecting the mid and apical LV segments, with preserved or hyperdynamic function of the basal segments, suggests Takotsubo cardiomyopathy (Table 3.1)[2, 3], especially in women aged >50 after an emotional shock.

2. Global systolic function

- Report global LV systolic function (Chapter 2).
- Report LV ejection fraction and LVOT velocity time integral, as both have important prognostic information.
- If the LV ejection fraction appears impaired by eye, measure systolic and diastolic volumes using biplane Simpson's method or 3D when available and feasible. The LV ejection fraction is used to guide medical treatment and the decision for biventricular pacing and/or defibrillator.

DOI: 10.1201/9781003242789-3

Table 3.1 Features of Takotsubo cardiomyopathy[3]

Transient hypokinesis, akinesis, or dyskinesis of the left ventricular mid-segments with or without apical involvement.
The regional wall motion abnormalities extend beyond a single epicardial vascular distribution.
Absence of significant obstructive coronary disease* or angiographic evidence of acute plaque rupture.
New electrocardiographic abnormalities (either ST-segment elevation and/or T wave inversion) or modest elevation in cardiac troponin.
Absence of phaeochromocytoma or myocarditis.

* May rarely coexist with obstructive coronary disease.

3. Right ventricle

- Assess RV size and regional and global systolic function (Chapter 4).
- Up to 30% of all inferior infarcts are associated with RV infarcts, and in 10%, the RV involvement is haemodynamically significant.
- Estimate pulmonary artery pressure (Chapter 5).

4. Describe the mitral valve

- Mitral regurgitation is common after myocardial infarction (Table 3.2).
- A restricted posterior leaflet causing a posteriorly directed jet is common after an inferior or inferolateral (posterior) infarction (Figure 3.1).
- 'Tenting' of both leaflets leading to a central jet occurs when there is dilatation of the mid and apical parts of the LV cavity (Figure 9.5, page 107).
- More complex situations can arise with restriction of some parts of the leaflet and prolapse of other parts. This can be secondary to stretching or rupture of minor chords or papillary muscle dysfunction.
- Grade the mitral regurgitation (Chapter 9, pages 114 and 115). Even moderate mitral regurgitation affects mortality independent of other factors[2] and may influence the decision to offer surgery rather than coronary angioplasty.
- 3D TTE and, occasionally, 2D/3D TOE may be required for the detailed evaluation of mitral valve morphology and the mechanism of regurgitation[4].

Table 3.2 Causes of mitral regurgitation after myocardial infarction

Restricted posterior mitral leaflet (Figure 3.1)
LV dilatation leading to symmetrical 'tenting' of the mitral leaflets
Rupture of major chords
Dysfunction or rupture of papillary muscle
Mitral prolapse secondary to minor chordal dysfunction
Coexistent primary mitral valve disease

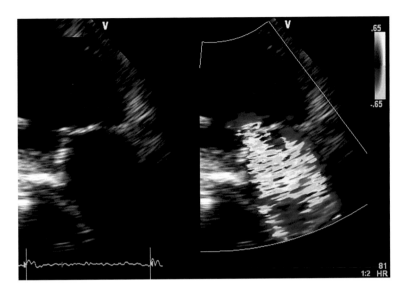

Figure 3.1 **Restricted posterior mitral leaflet.** Abnormal stresses on the posterior mitral leaflet as a result of an inferior or inferolateral myocardial infarct cause systolic restriction of the posterior leaflet (left), 'asymmetric tenting', with a posteriorly directed jet of regurgitation (right).

 And here's an electronic link to a loop on the website or use
http://goo.gl/B5lO2h

 And here's an electronic link to 3 or 4 loops on the website or use
http://goo.gl/txLqiv

Table 3.3 **Complications after myocardial infarction detected on TTE**[1]

True aneurysm (Figure 3.2a)	False aneurysm (Figure 3.2b)
Mitral regurgitation (Table 3.2)	Papillary muscle dysfunction/rupture
Ventricular septal rupture	Free-wall rupture ± tamponade
Thrombus (Table 18.6, page 206)	
Heart failure/cardiogenic shock*	Pericarditis*

* Clinical diagnosis supported by focused echocardiography.

5. **Complications** (Table 3.3)

- If there is a murmur, check for mitral regurgitation and ventricular septal rupture. These may occasionally coexist. Off-axis views are often necessary.
- A ventricular septal rupture may initially be obvious from abnormal systolic flow in the RV.

31

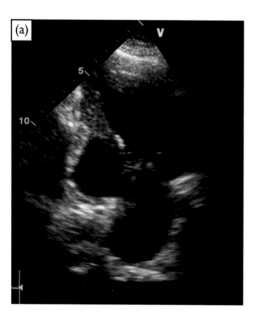
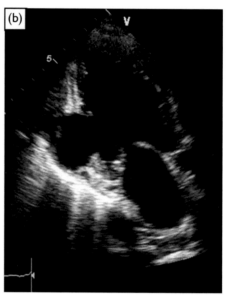

Figure 3.2 **True and false aneurysm.** A true aneurysm (a) is caused by the infarct bulging outwards so that there is a wide neck, and the myocardium is often seen in the border zone of the aneurysm. A false aneurysm (b) is a rupture of the infarcted myocardial wall with blood contained by the pericardium so that the false aneurysm contains no myocardial tissue.

 And here's an electronic link to a loop on the website or use http://goo.gl/wvoGQ4

- If there is mitral regurgitation, consider the causes in Table 3.2.
- All complications must be reported immediately to the clinician in charge of the case.
- A true aneurysm complicates about 5% of all anterior infarcts and is a sign of poor prognosis. It must be distinguished from a false aneurysm caused by free wall rupture contained by the pericardium (Table 3.4) (Figure 3.2).
- Occasionally, a true aneurysm leaks and is associated with a false aneurysm.
- Sometimes an aneurysm is found in the absence of an acute history. The differential diagnosis is given in Table 3.5.

6. Consider stress echocardiography

Indications for stress echocardiography in an acute coronary syndrome[1] include:

- Typical cardiac chest pain with normal or equivocal ECG changes (e.g. LBBB, RBBB, paced rhythm) and normal troponin levels.
- Normal or minimal troponin rise, but clinically stable, and high risk for contrast angiography (e.g. renal failure).

- Residual coronary stenosis in a non-culprit vessel, and decision for intervention to be based on ischaemic burden.
- Low-dose viability assessment if this will affect intervention.

Table 3.4 **Differentiation of true and false aneurysms**

	True aneurysm (Figure 3.2a)	False aneurysm (Figure 3.2b)
Position	More commonly apical	More commonly inferolateral
Neck	Commonly wide	Commonly narrow
Lining of aneurysm	Myocardium	Pericardium
Border zone	Gradually thinning myocardium stretching into the aneurysm	Punched-out edge to the myocardium
Colour flow	Absent or very slow flow	Into in systole, out in diastole

Table 3.5 **Differential diagnosis of apical aneurysm as a presenting feature**

Coronary disease
Syphilis
Chagas disease
Iatrogenic (e.g. surgical vent)
Congenital
Tuberculosis
Hypertrophic cardiomyopathy (Chapter 7, page 67)
Arrhythmogenic RV cardiomyopathy with LV involvement

 # MISTAKES TO AVOID

- Failing to detect secondary mitral regurgitation and to determine its aetiology.
- Missing inferior wall motion abnormalities with incomplete views.
- Missing a ventricular septal rupture by not using off-axis views.
- Not responding to a hyperdynamic LV, which may suggest a large ventricular septal rupture or severe mitral regurgitation.
- Not looking for the other cardiac causes of chest pain when the LV appears normal—aortic dissection and pulmonary embolism (Tables 19.2 and 19.5, pages 214 and 215).

CHECKLIST REPORT IN ACUTE CORONARY SYNDROME

1. LV size and function.
   a. Dimensions.
   b. Regional wall motion.
   c. Global systolic function.
2. Complications (Table 3.3), including mitral regurgitation grade and mechanism.
3. RV size, regional and global systolic function.
4. Estimated pulmonary artery systolic pressure.
5. Exclude other causes of acute chest pain, especially aortic dissection and acute pulmonary embolism.

References

1. Chatzizisisa YS, Venkatesh L, Murthyb VL & Solomona S. Echocardiographic evaluation of coronary artery disease. Coronary Artery Disease 2013;24:613–23.
2. Ghadri JR, Ruschitzka F, Luscher TF & Templin C. Takotsubo cardiomyopathy: Still much to learn. Heart 2014;100:1804–12.
3. Prasad A, Lerman A & Rihal CS. Apical ballooning syndrome (Tako-Tsubo or stress cardiomyopathy): A mimic of acute myocardial infarction. Am Heart J 2008;155:408–17.
4. Doherty JU, Kort S, Mehran R, Schoenhagen P & Soman P. ACC/AATS/AHA/ASE/ASNC/HRS/SCAI/SCCT/SCMR/STS 2019 appropriate use criteria for multimodality imaging in the assessment of cardiac structure and function in nonvalvular heart disease. J Am Coll Cardiol 2019;73:488–516.

- RV function affects prognosis in all types of cardio-pulmonary disease.
- A basic scan is done for suspected pulmonary embolism or in COVID-19 looking for RV dilatation.
- For a minimum standard study, the assessment includes:
  - Relative RV size in comparison with other cardiac chambers.
  - Measurement of the basal RV inflow diameter (RVD1 in Figure 4.1).
  - RV systolic function (TAPSE and DTI of TV annulus).

- A comprehensive assessment should be considered if it will change management and there is:
  - RV dilatation on the initial study
  - Congenital heart disease
  - Severe left-sided valve disease
  - Right-sided valve disease
  - Suspected RV cardiomyopathy
  - Pulmonary hypertension
  - Cardiac transplantation

1. **Is the RV dilated?**
   - Use multiple views optimised for the RV:
     - Parasternal long- and short-axis views at the aortic level for the measurement of RVOT diameter.
     - Parasternal short-axis views at basal, mid-, and apical RV levels (obtained at corresponding levels for the LV short-axis views).
     - The RV-focused apical 4-chamber view (Figure 4.1).
     - The RV is significantly dilated when it looks the same size or larger than the normal LV in the apical 4-chamber view (be careful when the left heart is also dilated).
     - As a guide, a diameter >41 mm at the base (RVD1) or >35 mm at the mid-level (RVD2) (Figure 4.1) in the RV-focused view indicates RV dilatation[1].
     - If the RV is dilated, multiple 2D diameters should be measured (Table 4.1), as explained in Figure 4.1.

     - The new NORRE recommendations[2, 3] are significantly different from the joint ASE/EACVI 2015 guidelines[1] (Table 4.1). The clinical implications have not been explored, but the ASE/EACVI 2015 values are still used for current guidelines on managing pathology, for example, ARVC.
     - **We suggest using the ASE/EACVI values until a consensus emerges.**

DOI: 10.1201/9781003242789-4

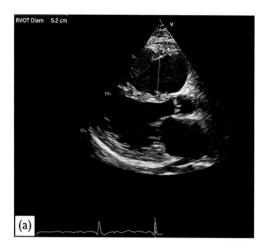

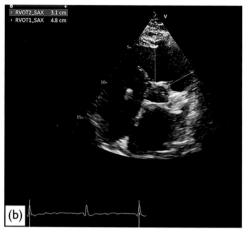

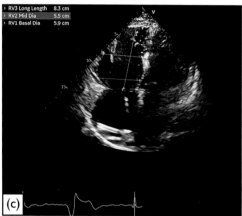

Figure 4.1 **2D RV measurements in ARVC/D.** These images show the recommended RV measurements in patients suspected of ARVC/D: (a) Dilated RVOT at 52 mm in PLAX view; (b) dilated RVOT in short-axis view, with proximal dimension at 48 mm and distal dimension at 31 mm; (c) dilated RV in apical 4-chamber view with RVD1 at 59 mm, RVD2 at 55 mm, and RV length at 83 mm.

Table 4.1 **Upper limit of normal RV dimensions (mm)**

RV dimensions	ASE/EACVI 2015[1]	NORRE[2, 3]	
		Male	Female
RVOT (P/S long-axis)	30	–	–
RVOT proximal (P/S short-axis)	35	44	42
RVOT distal (P/S short-axis)	27	29	28
Basal (RVD1)	41	47	43
Mid (RVD2)	35	42	35
Length base to apex (RVD3)	83	87	80
RV areas (cm²/m²)			
RVED area (men)	≤12.6	≤13.6	
RVED area (women)	≤11.5	≤12.6	

Table 4.2 **Suggested upper limit of normal for RV 3D volumes (mL/m²)[1]**

RV 3D volumes (mL/m²)	Male	Female
RVEDV	87	74
RVESV	44	36

- Take care in measuring RV end-systolic and end-diastolic measurements since major variability is caused by:
  - Failure to optimise the RV-focused apical views.
  - The presence of RV trabeculations and the moderator band.
  - Limited visualisation of the endocardium.
- Sex-specific values and BSA indexing of 2D-derived values are included in all recent recommendations[1–3] but are not routinely used in clinical practice.
- If the RV is confirmed as dilated on 2D linear measurements and systolic function is visually impaired, the measurement of RV volumes on 3D is recommended.
- Normal 3D echo values for RV volumes are still to be established in large population groups. The ASE/EACVI 2015 guidelines give the 3D RV upper volumes in Table 4.2.
- RV 3D volumes are lower than by CMR, but the RV ejection fraction is similar by both techniques[1].

2. **If dilated, is the RV active or hypokinetic?**
   - An active RV suggests volume overload caused by a left-to-right shunt at atrial level or significant tricuspid or pulmonary regurgitation (Table 4.3).

Table 4.3 **Causes of RV dilatation**

Active RV
Left-to-right shunt above the RV (e.g. ASD)
Severe tricuspid or pulmonary regurgitation
Hypokinetic RV
RV pressure overload: acute or chronic pulmonary embolism, congenital heart disease (with RV outflow obstruction), ARDS, severe left-sided heart disease
RV infarction
RV cardiomyopathy
End-stage pulmonary stenosis or regurgitation or tricuspid regurgitation
Post–cardiac surgery and lobectomy, pneumonectomy
Constrictive pericarditis and post-pericardiectomy

Table 4.4 **Thresholds for abnormal RV function**[1]

Tissue Doppler systolic velocity	<10 cm/s
TAPSE	<17 mm
RV FAC	<35%
RV 3D EF	<45%
RV free wall strain (research use)	>−19% (absolute value <19%)

- A hypokinetic RV suggests either pressure load or myocardial disease (Table 4.3).
- Look for RV regional wall motion abnormalities and always check the inferior wall of the LV, because about a third of inferior LV infarcts are associated with RV infarction.
- A dilated RV with regional wall motion abnormalities (+/– aneurysms), especially in the context of a family history of sudden cardiac death, suggests ARVC (see page 75).

3. **Quantification of RV systolic function** (Table 4.4)
   - **Tissue Doppler imaging** (TDI) measured as described in Figure 4.2a. An S′ velocity <10 cm/s indicates RV systolic dysfunction.
   - **TAPSE** (tricuspid annular plane systolic excursion) measured as described in Figure 4.2b. TAPSE <17 mm is abnormal.
   - **RV 2D fractional area change (FAC)** provides an estimate of global RV systolic function. This can be performed manually in the apical 4-chamber view but otherwise is generated automatically from the RV 3D data (Figure 4.3). RV FAC < 35% indicates RV systolic dysfunction[1].

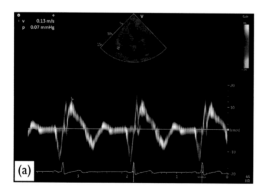
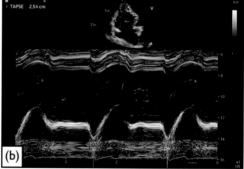

Figure 4.2 **Assessment of RV systolic function.** (a) Peak TDI systolic velocity of the tricuspid annulus. Place a pulsed Doppler tissue sample on the tricuspid annulus, ensuring good alignment with the RV free wall motion. Record the peak systolic velocity. (b) RV TAPSE. Place the M-mode cursor on the junction between the RV free wall and tricuspid annulus in a 4-chamber view. Ensure it is exactly aligned along the direction of the tricuspid lateral annulus, avoiding cutting through the RV basal lateral wall myocardium. Measure the excursion as the vertical distance between the peak and nadir.

- **RV 3D ejection fraction** (Figure 4.3)
  - May be useful after cardiac surgery (in the absence of marked septal shift), since conventional indices (TAPSE, S') are no longer representative.
  - As a guide, RV ejection fraction <45% suggests abnormal RV systolic function[1].

4. Is there RV hypertrophy?

- Defined by a free wall thickness >5 mm. This is best measured in the subcostal view level with the tips of the tricuspid valve.

- RV hypertrophy suggests:
  - Pulmonary hypertension (page 45).
  - Storage diseases—e.g. Fabry, Pompe.
  - Infiltrative diseases—e.g. amyloidosis.
  - Hypertrophic cardiomyopathy, Noonan's syndrome.

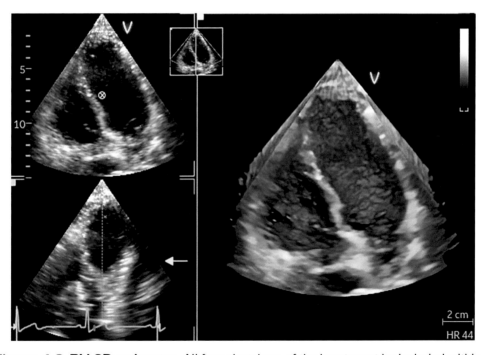

Figure 4.3 RV 3D volumes. All four chambers of the heart must be included within the pyramidal dataset to allow correct recognition of the RV. Use gated-acquisition full volume over four to six cardiac cycles for the best results. 3D data analysis is performed automatically and allows for manual correction of borders, both at end-diastole and systole. The analysis results include all RV apical linear dimensions, RV volumes, RV ejection fraction, FAC, and TAPSE from a single 3D volume dataset.

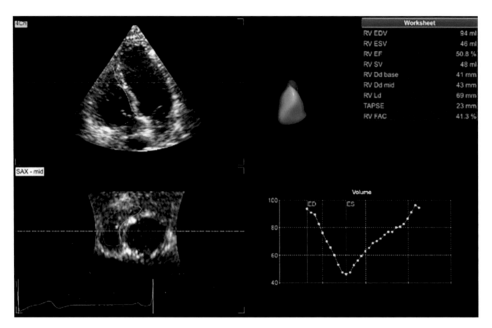

Worksheet	
RV EDV	94 ml
RV ESV	46 ml
RV EF	50.8 %
RV SV	48 ml
RV Dd base	41 mm
RV Dd mid	43 mm
RV Ld	69 mm
TAPSE	23 mm
RV FAC	41.3 %

Figure 4.3 (Continued)

5. **Is there left-sided disease?**
   - RV dilatation secondary to pulmonary hypertension may complicate severe mitral stenosis.
   - It can also occur in end-stage aortic stenosis and, occasionally, mitral regurgitation or severe LV dysfunction.

6. **Is there evidence of a shunt above the RV?**
   - If the RV is dilated and active but no ASD is visible, injection of agitated saline may help unmask it.
   - Otherwise, consider TOE, CMR, or CT to detect a sinus venosus defect or partial anomalous pulmonary venous drainage.

7. **Is there tricuspid and pulmonary regurgitation** (pages 121 and 125)?

8. **Estimate pulmonary artery pressure** (Chapter 5)

9. **Other imaging modalities:**
   - **CMR** is the gold standard technique for assessing RV volumes and should be considered for serial studies in patients with severe pulmonary regurgitation to guide the timing of intervention.

MISTAKES TO AVOID

- Overestimating RVOT dimensions by scanning from low parasternal positions.
- Foreshortening the RV by scanning from a rib space too high, which can lead to overestimating the transverse diameters.
- Including pericardial fat, trabeculations, or papillary muscles when measuring RV wall thickness.
- Incorrect cursor alignment to include the RV basal free wall adjacent to the tricuspid annulus when assessing TAPSE. This underestimates values.
- Including trabeculations, papillary muscles, and moderator band when tracing RV endocardium for measuring RV area or volume.

CHECKLIST REPORT FOR THE RV

1. RV size.
2. Global and regional RV systolic function.
3. Pulmonary pressures (Chapter 5).
4. Right-sided valve disease (Chapter 10).
5. Evidence of a shunt (Chapters 6 and 16).
6. Presence of left-sided disease.

References

1. Lang RM, Badano LP, MD, Mor-Avi V, et al. Recommendations for cardiac chamber quantification by echocardiography in adults: An update from the American Society of Echocardiography and the European Association of Cardiovascular Imaging. J Am Soc Echo 2015;28(1):1–39.
2. Lancellotti P, Badano LP, Lang RM, et al. Normal reference ranges for echocardiography: Rationale, study design, and methodology (NORRE Study). Europ Heart J CVI 2013;14(4):303–8.
3. Harkness A, Ring L, Augustine DX, et al. Guidelines and recommendations: Normal reference intervals for cardiac dimensions and function for use in echocardiographic practice: A guideline from the British Society of Echocardiography. Echo Research and Practice 2020;7(1):G1–18.

Pulmonary Pressure and Pulmonary Hypertension

5

- An elevated pulmonary artery (PA) systolic pressure is a marker of a poor clinical outcome, regardless of aetiology.
- The assessment of right-sided pressures is needed for two reasons:
  - The estimation of PA systolic pressure, where this is needed to aid clinical management, notably in mitral valve disease.
  - The detection of pulmonary hypertension.

Estimating PA Systolic Pressure

1. **Estimating the right ventricular (RV) to right atrial (RA) pressure difference**
   - Measure the TR V_{max}.
     - Ensure correct alignment with the direction of the jet.
     - Obtain a full Doppler envelope. Inspiratory hold or bubble contrast may be helpful for trivial jets of TR.
     - If the signal varies, take the highest value.
   - Estimate the RV–RA pressure difference ($4 \times$ TR V_{max})^2.
   - Estimate the RA pressure (see next section and Tables 5.1 and 5.2).
   - The sum of the RV–RA pressure difference and RA pressure gives an estimate of RV systolic pressure. This is the same as PA systolic pressure, assuming that there is no pulmonary stenosis or other RV outflow obstruction.

Table 5.1 **Estimating RA pressure[1]***

	Normal 0–5 mmHg Mean 3 mmHg	Intermediate 5–10 mmHg Mean 8 mmHg		High 10–20 mmHg Mean 15 mmHg
IVC diameter (mm)	≤21	≤21	>21	>21
Collapse with sniff	>50%	<50%	>50%	<50%

* Either a range or a mean value may be used, depending on local preference.

DOI: 10.1201/9781003242789-5

Table 5.2 **Secondary indices if the RA pressure estimate is intermediate**

Restrictive right-sided filling pattern (tricuspid E/A >2.1, deceleration time <120 ms)
Tricuspid E/E′ >6
Diastolic flow dominance in the hepatic vein
RA dilatation with no other cause (e.g. tricuspid regurgitation or atrial fibrillation)
Displacement of atrial septum to the left throughout the cycle

- This method has only moderate precision, and significant under- and overestimation can occur. The measurement of TR V_{max} should always be used in conjunction with other TTE markers of pulmonary hypertension[2, 3].
- In patients with severe free-flowing TR, the correlation between TR V_{max} and RV/PA systolic pressure is poor and an estimate should not be made.
- If there is any RV outflow obstruction (e.g. pulmonary stenosis), the RV systolic pressure will not reflect the PA systolic pressure. It is important to check the whole of the RV outflow (sub-pulmonary area, pulmonary valve, main and branch pulmonary arteries) for evidence of obstruction[4].
- Large left-to-right shunts (e.g. large VSD, aorto-pulmonary window, PDA) will cause equalization of RV/PA pressure with LV/aortic pressure. There is no need to measure the TR V_{max}, as it will just reflect the systemic systolic blood pressure[4].
- A VSD ejecting into the region of the tricuspid valve may 'contaminate' the spectral Doppler trace, making it uninterpretable[4].

2. **Estimating right atrial (RA) pressure**
- This is based on the diameter of the IVC (subcostal view) and response to a sniff (Tables 5.1 and 5.2).
  - The diameter should be measured at end expiration close to the junction with the hepatic veins 10–20 mm from the ostium of the RA.
  - Avoid the IVC moving out of the imaging plane during sniffing, which can exaggerate the reduction in diameter.
  - In acutely ill patients in whom the subcostal view is suboptimal, a right anterior oblique mid-axillary view can be used instead[5].
- Estimating RA pressure is semi-qualitative.

- When IVC diameter and response to a sniff are discordant (intermediate in Table 5.1):
  - Assign as 'high' if the IVC collapses <50%.
  - Assign as 'normal' if there are no secondary indices (Table 5.2).
  - Assign as 'intermediate' if the IVC collapses >50% but there are some secondary indices (Table 5.2).

3. Making the estimate of PA systolic pressure

RV systolic pressure is the sum of the RV–RA pressure difference plus the estimated RA pressure, provided there is no RV outflow obstruction.

- In mitral stenosis, a PA systolic pressure >50 mmHg at rest is an indication for balloon valvotomy, even in the absence of symptoms[6].
- In severe aortic stenosis (AS), a PA systolic pressure >60 mmHg indicates a high risk of dying, unless surgery or a TAVI is performed[6, 7].
  - This identifies the patient as having critical AS, meaning, that intervention is needed as soon as possible.
  - Inform the clinician in charge of the case.
- A rise in TR V_{max} is a secondary sign of deterioration in any type of valve disease and may aid the cardiologist to recommend intervention in otherwise-equivocal cases.

Assessing the Probability of Pulmonary Hypertension

- Pulmonary hypertension (PH) is defined as a mean pulmonary arterial pressure (mPAP) ≥25 mmHg at rest by right heart catheterization.
- However, the probability of PH can be estimated from the TR V_{max} at rest (Table 5.3).
- If the TR signal is not analysable, the signal may be improved by bubble contrast.

1. Estimating the probability of PH from the PA systolic signal

- A PA acceleration time >105 ms excludes pulmonary hypertension[10], and <80 ms makes pulmonary hypertension highly likely. This method is not accurate enough to give an estimate of absolute pressure (Figure 5.1a).

2. Estimating the probability of PH from the PR late-diastolic signal

- Optimise the continuous wave pulmonary regurgitant signal ideally to capture the full waveform.

Table 5.3 **Probability of PH based on TR V_{max}**

TR V_{max}	Probability of PH
≤2.8 m/s	Low
2.9–3.4 m/s	Check for other signs of PH (Figure 5.3)
>3.4 m/s	High

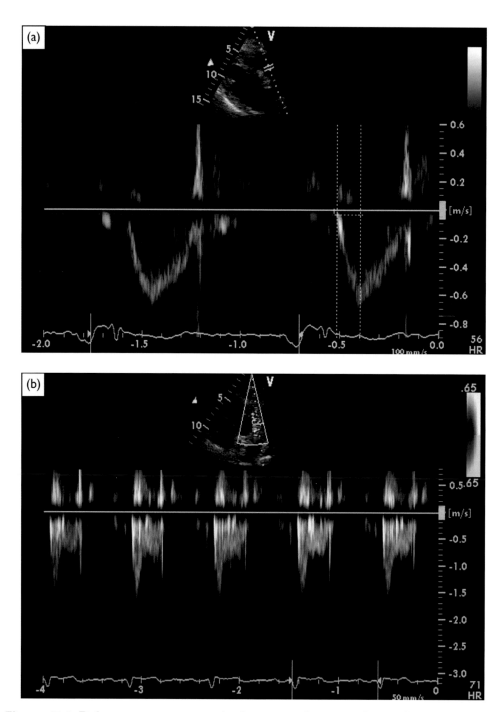

Figure 5.1 **Pulmonary artery velocity waveform and acceleration time.**
A normal waveform with time to peak velocity 120 ms (a) and a recording in a patient with
pulmonary hypertension (b). The time to peak velocity is short and the signal is notched
because of increased wave reflectance.

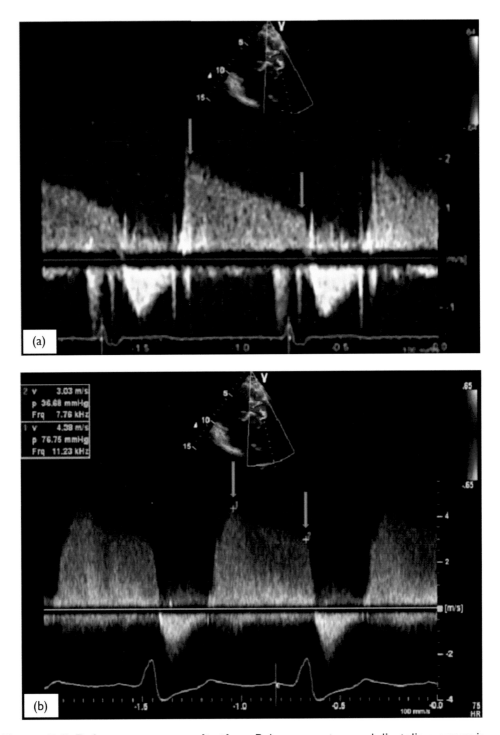

Figure 5.2 **Pulmonary regurgitation.** Pulmonary artery end-diastolic pressure is estimated using the end-diastolic velocity of the pulmonary regurgitant continuous wave signal (arrow) added to an estimate of RA pressure: (a) is a signal from a patient with a normal PA pressures, and (b) from a patient with pulmonary hypertension.

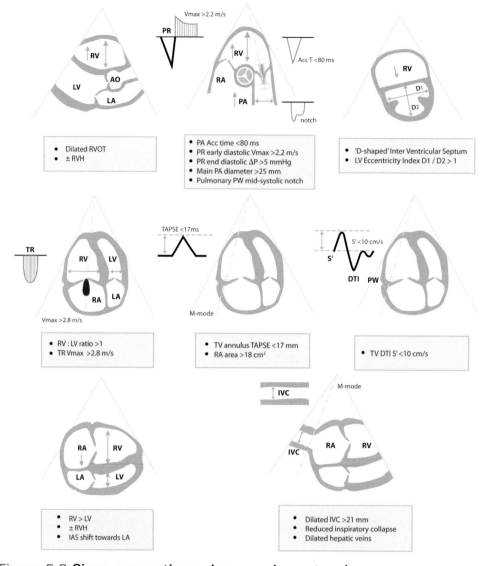

Figure 5.3 **Signs suggesting pulmonary hypertension.**

- Measure the end-diastolic velocity of the pulmonary regurgitant signal (Figure 5.2) and estimate the pressure difference ($4v^2$).
- An end-diastolic pressure difference >5 mmHg suggests PH[8].
- To estimate PA end-diastolic pressure:
  - Estimate the RA pressure (Tables 5.1 and 5.2).
  - End-diastolic PA pressure = PR end-diastolic pressure difference + RA pressure.

- This technique is not reliable if there is severe PR[4].

3. **Estimating the probability of PH from the PR early-diastolic signal**
   - Measure the peak velocity of the pulmonary regurgitant signal. A V_{max} >2.2 m/s suggests PH.
   - To estimate mean PA pressure:
     - Calculate the pressure difference ($4v^2$).
     - Estimate the RA pressure (Tables 5.1 and 5.2).
     - Mean PA pressure = PR peak diastolic pressure difference + RA pressure.
   - **A summary of signs suggesting pulmonary hypertension** is given in Figure 5.3.

4. **Assess RA and RV size and systolic function** (Chapters 4 and 6)
   - Flattening of the interventricular septum in systole causing a 'D-shaped' LV cavity is a clue that there could be PH.
   - An RA area >20 cm^2 is enlarged. One cause is PH.

5. **Look for causes of pulmonary hypertension**
   - The cardiac causes will be seen on TTE (Table 5.4).
   - Other causes may be suggested by the presence of valve thickening or regurgitation (e.g. SLE, antiphospholipid syndrome, anorexic drugs) or aortic dilatation (e.g. rheumatoid arthritis).

Table 5.4 **Cardiac causes of pulmonary hypertension detectable on TTE[9]**

Pulmonary venous hypertension
Valve disease • Mitral valve disease (stenosis > regurgitation) • Severe aortic stenosis (pulmonary hypertension in at least 25%)
Severe left ventricular impairment • Cardiomyopathy • LV failure of any cause
Congenital heart disease without shunts • Coarctation • Subaortic or supravalvar stenosis
Pericardial constriction
Left atrial obstruction • Myxoma • Cor triatriatum

(Continued)

Table 5.4 **Cardiac causes of pulmonary hypertension detectable on TTE**[9] (Continued)

Pulmonary venous hypertension (Continued)
Pulmonary vein obstruction • Congenital vein stenosis • Mediastinal pathology (fibrosis, tumour)
Chronic left-to-right shunts
ASD, VSD, patent ductus arteriosus, ruptured aortic sinus, aorto-pulmonary window

6. Confirming pulmonary hypertension

- Proving the diagnosis and grading the severity of PH requires a right heart catheter. The new haemodynamic definition of PH suggests a mPAP>20 mmHg and PVR 2 WU as a means of early detection.[11]

 # MISTAKES TO AVOID

- Overdiagnosis of pulmonary hypertension when screening patients. The TTE can only grade the probability of PH[2].
- Over-reliance on the TR V_{max}, which should always be used in conjunction with other TTE markers.
- Overdiagnosis. Pulmonary pressures increase with age and weight, so a pulmonary artery systolic pressure of 35–40 mmHg may be normal in an elderly or obese patient[1].
- Using IVC size and collapse in continuous mechanical ventilation since these are unreliable. The pressure from a central line should be used instead or judgements made using clinical observations.

CHECKLIST FOR REPORT IN PULMONARY HYPERTENSION

1. Estimated pulmonary pressures or presence/absence of pulmonary hypertension.
2. RV size and systolic function.
3. Tricuspid regurgitation grade.
4. Underlying cause.

References

1. McQuillan B, Picard M, Leavitt M & Weyman A. Clinical correlates and reference intervals for pulmonary artery systolic pressure among echocardiographically normal subjects. Circulation 2001;104(23):2797–802.
2. Augustine DX, Coates-Bradshaw LD, Willis J, et al. Echocardiographic assessment of pulmonary hypertension: A guideline protocol from the British Society of Echocardiography. Echo Res Pract 2018;5(3):G11–24.
3. Galie N, Humbert M, Vachieryc JL, et al. 2015 ESC/ERS guidelines for the diagnosis and treatment of pulmonary hypertension. Europ Heart J 2016;37(1):67–119.
4. Skinner GJ. Echocardiographic assessment of pulmonary arterial hypertension for pediatricians and neonatologists. Front Pediatr 2017;5:168.
5. Abbas AE, Fortuin FD, Schiller NB, Appleton CP, Moreno CA & Lester SJ. Echocardiographic determination of mean pulmonary artery pressure. Am J Cardiol 2003;92(11):1373–6.
6. Baumgartner H, Falk V, Bax JJ, et al. 2017 ESC/EACTS Guidelines for the management of valvular heart disease the task force for the management of valvular heart disease of the European Society of Cardiology (ESC) and the European Association for Cardio-Thoracic Surgery (EACTS). Europ Heart J 2017;38(36):2739–91.
7. Genereux P, Pibarot P, Redfors B, et al. Staging classification of aortic stenosis based on the extent of cardiac damage. Europ Heart J 2017;38(45):3351–8.
8. Ristow B, Ahmed S, Wang L, et al. Pulmonary regurgitation end-diastolic gradient is a Doppler marker of cardiac status: Data from the heart and soul study. J Am Soc Echocardiogr 2005;18(9):885–91.
9. McLaughlin VV, Atcher SL, Badesch DB, et al. ACCF/AHA 2009 expert consensus document on pulmonary hypertension. J Am Coll Cardiol 2009;53(17):1573–619.
10. Hoeper MM, Bogaard HJ, Condliffe R, et al. Definitions and diagnosis of pulmonary hypertension. J Am Coll Cardiol 2013;62(52):D42–50.
11. Humbert M, Kovacs G, Hoeper MM et al. 2022 ESC/ERS Guidelines for the diagnosis and treatment of pulmonary hypertension. Europ Heart J 2022;43(38):3618–3731.

The Atria and Atrial Septum

6

Left Atrium

- Left atrial (LA) size is not accurately represented by a linear dimension or area.
- Left atrial diameter (measured on 2D in a parasternal long-axis view) is still used:
  - In studies requested by electrophysiologists, since their literature still uses this dimension.
  - In hypertrophic cardiomyopathy, since the diameter is still part of the formula used to estimate the risk of sudden death[1].
- LA volume should always be measured in the following:
  - Systemic hypertension (as a sign of chronically increased filling pressure).
  - Atrial fibrillation (ant-post diameter and volume are both predictors of success of electrical cardioversion, catheter ablation of AF, and thromboembolic risk).
  - Suspected LV diastolic dysfunction.
  - Mitral valve disease (thromboembolic risk, indirect marker of severity).
  - Helping to discriminate an athletic heart from early cardiomyopathy (see Chapter 7).
- Measuring LA volume:
  - Planimeter the LA in optimised left atrial 4-chamber and 2-chamber views, excluding the pulmonary veins and appendage. Use Simpson's method. Index to BSA if BMI <30 kg/m^2.

Table 6.1 **Upper limits of normal for left atrial size[2, 3]**

		Males	Females
Ant-post dimension	Absolute (mm)	43.3	40.6
	Indexed (mm/m^2)	22.7	24.0
Area	Absolute (cm^2)	20.3	22.0
	Indexed (cm^2/m^2)	11.9	12.7
Volume*	Indexed (mL/m^2)	34	34

Note: Ant-post dimension measured in the anteroposterior plane in the parasternal long-axis view. Area at end-systole in the apical 4-chamber view. Volume by Simpson's biplane method at end-systole in the apical 4- and 2-chamber views. Upper limit of normal (ULN) based on mean + 2 SD.

* ULN for indexed volume based upon expert consensus[3], and corresponding absolute data not available.

DOI: 10.1201/9781003242789-6

- The upper limit of normal is 34 mL/m^2 [2, 3].
- Where suboptimal image quality permits measurement in only one plane, values tend to be 1–2 mL/m^2 smaller than the biplane equivalent. There are no normal ranges for 3D LA measurements yet[2].

- If there is a left atrial mass, see Chapter 18.

Right Atrium

- Right atrial area is measured in the minimum standard TTE. This is particularly important if:
  - It looks larger than the LA in the 4-chamber view.
  - There is atrial fibrillation (likely success of cardioversion, thromboembolic risk).
  - There is suspected RV or LV dysfunction.
  - There is pulmonary hypertension.
  - There is an ASD.
  - There is tricuspid valve disease.

- Image the right atrium in the right heart apical 4-chamber view at end-systole.
- Volume can be measured using the single-plane Simpson's method. Area is then given automatically (Table 6.2).
- Atrial dilatation can give a clue to the diagnosis (Table 6.3).
- If there is a mass, see Chapter 18.

Atrial Septum

1. **Is the septum thickened?**
   - Lipomatous hypertrophy is usually normal and occurs in a dumb-bell-shaped distribution, sparing the fossa ovalis in the middle.
   - An attached mass suggests a myxoma or, less commonly, a thrombus caught in a PFO.

Table 6.2 Upper limits of normal for right atrial size[3, 4]*

	Male	Female
Area (cm^2)	21.9	19.0
Indexed area (cm^2/m^2)	11.1	11.0
Volume (mL)	70.6	55.3
Volume (mL/m^2)	35.5	31.4

* Although this is the most contemporaneous data range for the RA, it was measured using a normal apical 4-chamber view. The upper limit is calculated as mean + 2 SD.

Table 6.3 **Causes of atrial enlargement**

Characteristically biatrial enlargement
Chronic atrial fibrillation
Restrictive cardiomyopathy
Rheumatic disease affecting mitral and tricuspid valves
Athletic heart (mild enlargement)
Pericardial constriction (mild or moderate enlargement)
Predominantly LA enlargement
Mitral stenosis or regurgitation
Left ventricular diastolic dysfunction
Predominantly RA enlargement
Tricuspid stenosis or regurgitation
Pulmonary hypertension
ASD
RV cardiomyopathy

2. **Is the septum mobile or aneurysmal?**
    - An atrial septal aneurysm is defined[5] (Figure 6.1) by:
        - A mobile segment with base >10 mm wide.
        - Excursion ≥10 mm between left and right atrium during spontaneous respiration.
    - A mobile septum is defined by an excursion of <10 mm and has no pathological significance.
    - An aneurysmal septum is often associated with a PFO. The presence of both together is associated with a significantly higher recurrence rate after cardioembolic stroke than with either alone[6].
    - Bowing of the whole septum may also occur as a result of severe TR or MR or high RA or LA pressures.
    - Sometimes, the aneurysm is fixed.

3. **ASD or dropout?**
    - In the 4-chamber view, it is common to see dropout. The uncertainty is usually resolved on other views and by the absence of abnormal flow on colour mapping.
    - If doubt remains, consider:
        - A saline contrast injection, which may make the ASD obvious as a void.

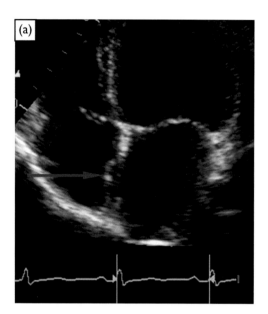
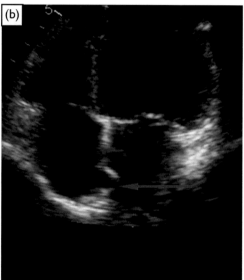

Figure 6.1 **Atrial septal aneurysm.** Maximum rightward (a) and leftward (b) extent.

- Pulsed Doppler on the RA side of the septum. ASD flow has a peak in late diastole and systole. For the superior vena cava, the peaks are earlier.
- TOE or CMR: TOE gives superior imaging of the interatrial septum and any defects. CMR provides accurate shunt quantification and accurate ventricular volumes.

4. Is there a PFO?

- These occur on bubble contrast TTE in c15% of the normal population[7] but may be more common and larger in:
  - Young people with TIA or cerebral infarcts.
  - Decompression sickness in divers.
  - Disproportionate hypoxia in critically ill patients.
  - The rarely seen patients who are normal lying down but become breathless, with a drop in oxygen saturation, when they stand up (platypnoea-orthodeoxia syndrome)[8].
- A PFO may be seen on colour imaging, most frequently in a subcostal view, with the colour scale reduced to maximise detection of low-velocity flow.
- More usually, a bubble study is needed (Table 6.4). This is usually better performed on TTE than TOE, since a Valsalva manoeuvre is easier in the conscious patient. A PFO is usually taken to be present if bubbles appear in the LA within three or fewer cardiac cycles after the contrast enters the RA.

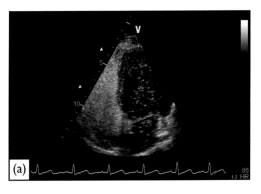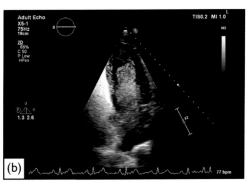

Figure 6.2 **Bubble contrast study.** These show a moderate (a) and large PFO (b).

Table 6.4 **Performing a bubble contrast study**

Allow adequate time. Practice the Valsalva manoeuvre at the start, ensuring that image quality is minimally affected and there is good leftward deviation of the atrial septum.
Ask the patient to breathe out then hold the breath and strain with the abdomen against a closed glottis with minimal movement of the chest. Practice instant release.
Place a 21 G cannula in an antecubital fossa vein and connect to a three-way tap.
Fill a syringe with about 8.5 mL 0.9% saline. For each injection, leave approximately 0.5 mL air in the syringe and withdraw approximately 1 mL venous blood into the syringe.
Attach a dry syringe to the other port of the three-way tap and agitate between the two syringes until a dense, uniform froth containing no large air bubbles is produced.
For the initial injections, there may be no manoeuvre. With the Valsalva manoeuvre, the injection should be timed to reach the right heart at release.
Other manoeuvres are asking the patient to cough or take a sharp sniff on right heart opacification.
Multiple injections with Valsalva should be given until attaining at least one with perfect synchronisation of all elements. Sometimes, several (up to 6) are necessary.
Archive about eight to ten cycles capturing the contrast arriving in the right heart and at least five cycles after this.

Table 6.5 Suggested methods of grading a patent foramen ovale[9]

Small	A small number of individual bubbles
Moderate	A few bubbles, but not sufficient to cause a bolus within the left atrium or to fill the whole of the left heart (Figure 6.2a)
Large	Left atrial bolus of bubbles too numerous to count or bubbles filling the whole of the left heart (Figure 6.2b)

- Grading a PFO is controversial and subjective:
  - Many thresholds for a large shunt appear in the literature based on the number of bubbles crossing to the LA.
  - However, counting individual bubbles is not usually easy in practice. We use the grading system in Table 6.5[9].
  - Individual studies should be discussed at an MDT concerning possible closure.

- Pulmonary arteriovenous malformations are suggested by[10, 11]:
  - Bubbles appearing after three cycles.
  - Bubbles entering via the pulmonary veins.
  - Slow clearance of the bubbles because of continuing replenishment.

 MISTAKES TO AVOID

- Overdiagnosing atrial dilatation from a diameter in one plane.
- Missing LA dilatation by measuring only an anteroposterior dimension without volume assessment.
- Failing to coordinate a Valsalva manoeuvre and the timing of the contrast injection when looking for a PFO.
- Mistaking SVC flow for an ASD.

CHECKLIST FOR REPORTING THE ATRIA

1. Sizes of LA and RA.
2. If LA or RA dilated, is there an obvious cause (Table 6.3)?
3. Appearance of atrial septum.
4. Is there evidence of a shunt?

References

1. O'Mahony C, Jichi F, Pavlou M, et al. A novel clinical risk prediction model for sudden cardiac death in hypertrophic cardiomyopathy (HCM risk-SCD). Eur Heart J 2014;35(30):2010–20.

2. Lang RM, Badano LP, Mor-avi V, et al. Recommendations for cardiac chamber quantification by echocardiography in adults : An update from the American Society of Echocardiography and the European Association of Cardiovascular Imaging. J Am Soc Echocardiogr 2015;28(1):1–39.

3. Harkness A, Ring L, Augustine DX, et al. Normal reference intervals for cardiac dimensions and function for use in echocardiographic practice: A guideline from the British Society of Echocardiography. Echo Res Pract 2020;7(1):G1–18.

4. Kou S, Caballero L, Dulgheru R, et al. Echocardiographic reference ranges for normal cardiac chamber size: Results from the NORRE study. Eur Heart J CVI 2014;15(6):680–90.

5. Gondi B, Nanda N. Two-dimensional echocardiographic features of atrial septal aneurysms. Circulation 1981;63(2):452–7.

6. Snijder RJR, Luermans JGLM, de Heij AH, et al. Patent foramen ovale with atrial septal aneurysm is strongly associated with migraine with aura: A large observational study. J Am Heart Assoc 2016;5(12):1–7.

7. Rundek T, Elkind MSV, Di Tullio MR, et al. Patent foramen ovale and migraine: A cross-sectional study from the Northern Manhattan Study (NOMAS). Circulation 2008;118(14):1419–24.

8. Cheng TO. Mechanisms of platypnea-orthodeoxia: What causes water to flow uphill? Circulation 2002;105(6):e47.

9. Chambers J, Seed PT & Ridsdale L. Association of migraine aura with patent foramen ovale and atrial septal aneurysms. Int J Cardiol. 2013;168(4):3949–53.

10. Rana BS, Thomas MR, Calvert PA, et al. Echocardiographic evaluation of patent foramen ovale prior to device closure. J Am Coll Cardiol CVI 2010;3(7):749–60.

11. Freeman JA & Woods TD. Use of saline contrast echo timing to distinguish intracardiac and extracardiac shunts: failure of the 3- to 5-beat rule. Echocardiography 2008;25(10):1127–30.

Cardiomyopathies 7

- Cardiomyopathies are heart muscle diseases not caused by pressure or volume overload or coronary artery disease[1-3].
- They may be caused by primary familial (genetic) muscle disease, by infiltrative processes (e.g. amyloid), by storage diseases (e.g. Fabry disease), or by external agents (e.g. alcohol, radiation, anthracyclines).
- Their diagnosis is based on a balance of clinical factors (presentation, family history, past medical history, examination), the ECG findings, and imaging.
- TTE is the first-line imaging technique and initially categorises as:
  - Dilated LV, including dilated cardiomyopathy (DCM).
  - Hypertrophied LV, including hypertrophic cardiomyopathy (HCM).
- Specific cardiomyopathies also have characteristic TTE features:
  - Restrictive cardiomyopathy—non-dilated LV and RV with high filling pressures and biatrial enlargement.
  - Non-compaction—hypertrabeculation.
  - Arrhythmogenic ventricular cardiomyopathy—RV dilatation, wall motion abnormalities, +/– LV involvement.

The Dilated LV

- Secondary myocardial impairment and dilated cardiomyopathies may look similar on TTE, but there may be clues to the aetiology (Table 7.1).

1. **LV size and systolic function**
   - Is the LV large? Borderline cavity dimensions and volumes should be indexed to BSA (Table 2.1, page 16).
   - Is the LV hypokinetic (Table 7.1), normal, or hyperkinetic (Table 7.2)? Borderline hypokinesis is normal in athletic hearts (Table 7.3).

2. **General appearance**
   - Is there a regional abnormality suggesting an ischaemic aetiology (Figure 2.4)?
   - Are both ventricles dilated, suggesting a cardiomyopathy?
   - Is there concentric LV hypertrophy, suggesting hypertension?
   - Is there a valve abnormality which might have caused the myocardial impairment?

DOI: 10.1201/9781003242789-7

Table 7.1 **Causes of a dilated, hypokinetic LV**

Common non-DCM cause	
Coronary artery disease	Regional wall abnormalities corresponding to coronary territories
Pressure overload Hypertension, severe AS	LVH, dilated aorta
Volume overload End-stage MR, AR	Differentiating secondary from primary MR may be difficult (see Chapter 9)
Renal failure	LVH, valve calcifications, pericardial effusion
DCM of acquired aetiology	
Tachyarrhythmia	Uncontrolled atrial tachyarrhythmia Very frequent ventricular ectopics
Alcohol	May recover after alcohol cessation in 50%
Drugs	Chemotherapeutic agents, verapamil, cocaine
Autoimmune systemic diseases Churg–Strauss syndrome Systemic lupus erythematous (SLE)	Impaired LV relaxation, MR, pericardial effusion Valve thickening, non-bacterial Libman–Sacks vegetations, pulmonary hypertension, pericardial effusion
Sarcoidosis	Thinning and dilatation crossing arterial territories
Peripartum cardiomyopathy	Last month of pregnancy and up to the first five months after delivery
Haemochromatosis (genetic disorder of iron metabolism)	Early diastolic dysfunction with raised filling pressures and dilated LA Arrhythmias (AF, VF)
Thalassaemia (inherited haemoglobin disorder)	Biventricular DCM, restrictive filling (iron overload), pulmonary hypertension
Uncommon causes	HIV (10% of asymptomatic cases), nutritional (thiamine), metabolic (hypothyroidism)
Post myocarditis DCM	
Viral Other vasculitis—Kawasaki	LV and RV increased wall thickness Dilated and aneurysmal coronary arteries, LV regional wall motion abnormalities

Table 7.1 (Continued)

Genetically determined DCM (family history of HF, CM, SCD)	
Muscular dystrophies Duchenne and Becker muscular dystrophy **LMNA cardiomyopathy**	Inferolateral akinesia AV block, ventricular arrhythmias
Idiopathic DCM	
Unknown aetiology	After excluding genetic factors
Specific preclinical DCM (new categories)[4]:	
Arrhythmic DCM	Familial history of SCD, ventricular arrhythmias
Hypokinetic non-DCM	Normal size, hypokinetic LV, severe diastolic dysfunction

Table 7.2 **Causes of a dilated, hyperkinetic LV**

Valve disease
Severe aortic regurgitation
Severe mitral regurgitation
Moderate or worse mixed aortic and mitral regurgitation
Shunts
Ventricular septal defect
Ruptured sinus of Valsalva aneurysm
Persistent ductus

Table 7.3 **Features of an athletic heart[5, 6]**

Increased LV end-diastolic diameter (rarely >60 mm) may persist for >5 years after stopping training. If associated with reduced LV ejection fraction and abnormal diastolic function, suggests DCM.
Normal systolic function, occasionally borderline global hypokinesis.
Mild left ventricular hypertrophy, septum usually ≤13 mm.
Normal LV diastolic function.
Mild RV dilatation and hypertrophy.

Table 7.4 **Echocardiographic findings in sarcoid[7]***

Dilated LV with global systolic dysfunction Regional wall motion abnormalities not in a coronary artery distribution Thin walls, most commonly the basal anterior septum (occasionally thickened in early disease, becoming thin later) LV aneurysms
Diastolic dysfunction—initially delayed relaxation, restrictive pattern in advanced disease
Focal intracardiac mass caused by a large granuloma that may involve papillary muscle, causing mitral regurgitation
RV dysfunction secondary to pulmonary disease
Pericardial effusion

* Multisystem disorder characterised by the growth of tiny collections of inflammatory cells (granulomas). High incidence of arrhythmias (AV block, BBB, SVT, VT) and SCD.

- Are there unusual features?
  - Regional wall motion abnormalities crossing arterial territories (e.g. sarcoid) (Table 7.4).
  - Bright endocardial echoes (e.g. haemochromatosis).
  - Apical echogenicity (consider thrombus, HCM, or non-compaction).
  - Abnormal myocardial density (non-specific, but consider amyloid).

3. **Quantify LV systolic function and assess LV diastolic function**
    See pages 20–25

4. **Are there complications?**
    - LV thrombus
    - Secondary mitral regurgitation (Table 7.5)
    - Pulmonary hypertension (see Chapter 5)

5. **Other imaging modalities:**
    - **CMR[8]:**
      - Differentiation of ischaemia from other causes of LV dilatation by the pattern of late gadolinium enhancement (transmural, patchy subendocardial, global subendocardial, epicardial, mid-wall).
      - Assessment of viability in ischaemic cardiomyopathy.
      - Better than TTE for LV morphology, volumes, and ejection fraction if image quality suboptimal.
      - May help the diagnosis of myocarditis using T1 and T2-weighted imaging to evaluate myocardial inflammation and oedema, and gadolinium enhancement to assess diseased myocardium.

Table 7.5 **Differentiating primary and secondary mitral regurgitation with a dilated LV**

Favours secondary regurgitation
Mitral valve normal in appearance, with dilated annulus
Mitral valve tented
Review of echocardiograms showing LV function declining while mitral regurgitation still mild
Favours primary regurgitation
Mitral valve abnormal in appearance (prolapsing, flail leaflet, or rheumatic)
Review of TTE shows severe mitral regurgitation with previously hyperdynamic LV

- T2* imaging detects and quantifies iron deposits in the myocardium in haemochromatosis.
- Detection of aneurysms in Chagas disease.

- **CT coronary angiography**: to look for coronary disease as a cause of LV dilatation. Especially used instead of invasive coronary angiography in young patients at low clinical risk of coronary disease.
- **Invasive contrast coronary angiography**: to look for coronary disease as a cause of LV dilatation, especially in patients at high or intermediate risk of coronary disease.
- **PET**: to identify myocardial viability.

MISTAKES TO AVOID

- Measuring LV obliquely, causing overdiagnosis of LV dilatation.
- Overdiagnosis of dilatation by not correcting for BSA in large individuals.
- Misdiagnosis of athlete's heart as cardiomyopathy.
- Mistaking LV dilatation caused by primary mitral valve disease as cardiomyopathy.

The Hypertrophied LV

- The cause of LV hypertrophy may be obvious if there is aortic stenosis or systemic hypertension.
- Often, it may be difficult to differentiate the effects of hypertension from an athletic heart or hypertrophic cardiomyopathy or less-common causes (Table 7.6).

Table 7.6 **Causes of increased LV wall thickness**[9,10]

Common		
Hypertension		
Aortic stenosis		
Renal disease		
African/Afro-Caribbean ethnicity		
Obesity		
Athletes (usually mild hypertrophy)		
Cardiomyopathies		
Hypertrophic cardiomyopathies (sarcomere)		
Metabolic genetic errors (storage disorders)	Glycogen storage diseases (e.g. Pompe, Danon)	
	Lysosomal storage diseases (e.g. Anderson–Fabry)	
	Carnitine disorders	
	AMP-kinase (PRKAG2)	
Infiltrative disorders—amyloidosis (familial ATTR, senile TTR, AL)		
Neuromuscular disease (e.g. Friedreich's ataxia)		
Malformation syndromes: Noonan, LEOPARD, Costello		
Mitochondrial diseases		
Drug-induced (e.q. tacrolimus, hydroxychloroquine, steroids)		

1. **Describe the pattern of hypertrophy**
   - Is it symmetrical or asymmetrical (Figure 2.2)?
   - Does it affect RV as well as LV? Symmetrical LV and RV hypertrophy suggests an infiltrative cardiomyopathy.
   - Asymmetrical hypertrophy usually suggests HCM. Describe its distribution, for example:
     - Septal hypertrophy (reverse curvature).
     - Apical (Figure 7.1).
     - Septum and free wall, with sparing of the posterior wall.
     - Papillary muscles hypertrophy +/– antero-apical displacement, double-bifid papillary, direct insertion into the MV leaflets.
     - Sigmoid septum or subaortic septal bulge. This is common in elderly patients. It may be the first site of hypertrophy associated with hypertension. If severe and in a young person with a family history, it may also be consistent with HCM.

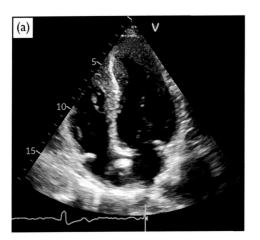
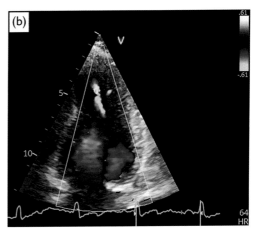

Figure 7.1 **Apical hypertrophic cardiomyopathy.** (a) Distal LV hypertrophy involving apical segments; (b) LV apical colour flow acceleration.

2. **If the hypertrophy is asymmetric, measure wall thickness at all levels.**
   - Measurements should initially be made in short-axis views perpendicular to the circumference of the endocardium and epicardium.
   - Exclude aberrant tendons and LV papillary muscles, RV papillary muscles, or moderator band.
   - Report the maximal wall thickness since this is used in the score to estimate the risk of sudden cardiac death in HCM. A wall thickness ≥30 mm in any segment is a strong marker of sudden death.
   - Measurements should be interpreted in the clinical context[10]:
     - In first-degree relatives (50% risk of inheritance), maximal wall thickness ≥13 mm is diagnostic of HCM.
     - Apical hypertrophy ≥13 mm associated with marked T wave inversion on the ECG is diagnostic of apical HCM.
     - Wall thickness ≥15 mm in a young patient with abnormal ECG and no previous medical history has a high probability of HCM. Exceptions occur, for example, Afro-Caribbean athletes.
     - Concentric hypertrophy 15–20 mm in African or Afro-Caribbean people may be secondary to hypertension.

3. **Quantify LV systolic and diastolic function.**
   - In HCM, LV radial systolic function is often preserved or increased, but longitudinal systolic function is frequently impaired (GLS > −15%).
   - A reduced LV ejection fraction <50% in HCM indicates a high risk for sudden cardiac death.
   - Impaired LV systolic function with significant concentric hypertrophy suggests amyloid rather than HCM.

- In end-stage 'burnt-out' HCM, the LV may be dilated and hypokinetic, with only mild hypertrophy. Review of older studies will validate the diagnosis.
- Impaired relaxation and pseudo-normal filling are the most common patterns of diastolic dysfunction in HCM. Restrictive physiology may be seen in advanced HCM but is more suggestive of amyloid.

4. **Is there an apical aneurysm?**
    - Aneurysm formation (+/– thrombus) is uncommon in HCM (2% in HCM; 13–15% in apical HCM) but indicates a high risk for sudden death[11].
    - Contrast TTE or sometimes CMR are needed if image quality is suboptimal.

5. **Measure LA size**
    - Measure LA linear dimension at end-systole in a 2D parasternal long-axis view. This is used to calculate the risk of sudden cardiac death.
    - Measure LA volume indexed to BSA (ideally on 3D, if available).
    - LA dilatation (LA volume >34 mL/m^2; LA diameter >48 mm) predicts sudden cardiac death[12] and indicates an increased risk of thromboembolism.

6. **Is there intra-LV or LVOT flow acceleration?**
    - Use colour and pulsed Doppler to locate the area of maximal flow acceleration. Use CW Doppler to record the maximal velocity.
    - Use pulsed Doppler to measure LVOT velocity at rest and CW if abnormal.
    - Use CW before and after a Valsalva manoeuvre performed semi-supine then sitting and, if no obstruction is provoked, on standing[9,10].
    - The measured peak LVOT gradient is used in the risk calculator of sudden cardiac death. In addition:
        - A peak gradient >50 mmHg, in symptomatic patients, is a threshold for myomectomy or alcohol ablation.
        - In patients with symptoms and resting or provoked LVOT gradient <50 mmHg, consider exercise testing[10] to look for worsening LVOT acceleration.

7. **Differential diagnosis of LVOT obstruction**
    - Look at the aortic valve and rule out AS or subaortic membrane as a cause of LV hypertrophy and LV obstruction.
    - Systolic anterior motion of the anterior mitral leaflet (SAM) causes a dynamic, late-systolic peak velocity.
    - AS and subaortic membrane cause a fixed obstruction with a velocity peak in early or mid-systole.
    - Do not forget the other haemodynamic and morphological changes that can cause SAM and LVOT obstruction (Table 7.7). These can lead to an overdiagnosis of HCM.

Table 7.7 **Non-HCM SAM and LVOT obstruction**

Haemodynamic changes	Causes
Decreased preload	Hypovolaemia
Increased LV inotropy	Fever, anaemia, inotropic drugs (e.g. dobutamine)
Morphological changes	Causes
Sigmoid septum	Hypertension, elderly heart
Acute coronary syndromes	Compensatory hyperkinesis of basal segments
Takotsubo cardiomyopathy	Catecholamine effect
Post–mitral valve repair	Annuloplasty ring with change in MV leaflet geometry
Transcatheter mitral valve in ring implant	Change in native MV leaflet orientation into LVOT

8. Assess the valves

Mitral valve:

- Look for SAM of the MV leaflets or of the chords alone.
- SAM more often involves the anterior leaflet but may occasionally affect the posterior leaflet alone or, more rarely, both.
- Is SAM incomplete or complete (leaflet contacts the septum)?
- Mitral regurgitation is mostly directed posteriorly away from the point of anterior motion but, in some cases, could be central or anteriorly directed.
- **Abnormal mitral valve appearance:**
  - Abnormally long anterior mitral valve leaflet (>16 mm).
  - Mitral valve thickening from septal contact (with mirror thickening of the basal septal endocardium).
  - Associated intrinsic MV disease like mitral prolapse may be present.
  - Evidence of previous endocarditis (HCM is a risk factor).

- **Abnormal mitral valve sub-apparatus:**
  - Papillary muscle hypertrophy.
  - Antero-apical displacement of the papillary muscles.
  - Double-bifid papillary muscles.
  - Direct insertion of MV leaflets into the papillary muscles.
  - Aberrant mitral valve chordae extending into LVOT.

Other valves:

- Mid-systolic closure of the aortic valve indicates LVOT obstruction.
- Look for sub-pulmonary valve stenosis, frequently seen in Noonan syndrome.
- Measure tricuspid regurgitation velocity and estimated pulmonary systolic pressure (see Chapter 6).

9. **Hypertrophic cardiomyopathy (HCM) vs hypertension**
   - The diagnosis of cardiomyopathy is made using all available clinical data.
   - The TTE alone should never be used to make a new diagnosis but can suggest HCM (Table 7.8).

10. **Hypertrophic cardiomyopathy (HCM) vs athletic heart**
    - Endurance or resistance training usually causes an increase in cavity size, but only mild septal thickening (≤13 mm) (Table 7.9).

11. **Hypertrophic cardiomyopathy (HCM) vs phenocopies**
    - HCM (sarcomeric) and phenocopies cannot be reliably differentiated based on imaging alone.
    - It is crucial to distinguish and correctly diagnose HCM phenocopies at an early stage, because prognosis and management differ significantly from HCM.
    - Table 7.10 shows features suggestive of HCM phenocopies.

Table 7.8 Features in favour of HCM rather than hypertensive disease

Asymmetrical hypertrophy most frequently affecting the septum
Hypertrophy affecting both ventricles
Septal hypertrophy ≥15 mm (Caucasian) and ≥20 mm (African/Afro-Caribbean)
Abnormally long mitral valve leaflet
Complete systolic anterior motion of the anterior mitral leaflet and severe LVOT flow acceleration (both may also be present in hypertension with sigmoid septum)
Severe diastolic dysfunction
No regression in hypertrophy after good blood pressure control
Large QRS voltages and T wave changes on ECG
Family history of HCM

Table 7.9 Features in favour of cardiomyopathy rather than athletic heart[5, 6, 10]

Asymmetric hypertrophy mainly affecting septum
Wall thickness: • >15 mm or 13–15 mm with no change after three months' detraining.   • In athletic heart (power athletes), the wall thickness is usually ≤12 mm.
Involvement of both RV as well as LV.

Table 7.9 (Continued)

LV cavity dimension <45 mm.
Significant LA enlargement. In athletic heart, there is mild LA enlargement.
Early markers of LV systolic dysfunction: • TDI S' <9 cm/s and reduced GLS. • In athletic heart, the LV ejection fraction may be low at rest, but TDI S' >9 cm/s and GLS normal.
Diastolic dysfunction E/A <1, prolonged E deceleration time, and low E'. In athletic heart, diastole is normal or supranormal, E/A >2, A velocity is low, E' lateral and septal increased, and E/E' low.
Associated SAM or mid-systolic aortic valve closure.
Eccentric RV remodelling particularly involving RV inflow tract. ARVC involves both inflow and outflow.
Female gender or family history of hypertrophic cardiomyopathy.
Abnormal ECG.

Table 7.10 **Features in favour of HCM phenocopies**

Diagnoses	TTE features[9, 10]
Cardiac amyloidosis	Concentric LVH Ground-glass appearance of the myocardium Thickened valves and interatrial septum Thickened RV wall Markedly reduced GLS with apical sparing Low ECG voltages Pericardial effusion
Fabry disease	LV hypertrophy mostly symmetrical, but may be asymmetrical Global hypokinesia +/− dilated LV Inferolateral mid-wall scarring Thickened valves Thickened RV wall
Danon, Pompe	Extreme concentric LVH
Noonan syndrome	RV hypertrophy with RVOT obstruction

Other imaging modalities:

CMR may be used to:
- Improve the description of the hypertrophy, particularly looking for RV involvement and apical LV involvement
- Identify LV apical aneurysms +/− thrombus
- Detect and quantify myocardial fibrosis
- Exclude differential diagnoses (amyloid, Anderson–Fabry, myocarditis)

MISTAKES TO AVOID

- Making a new diagnosis of HCM from the TTE alone. This is a clinical diagnosis based on past medical and family history, blood tests and ECG, genetic screening, and CMR.
- Incorrect measurements of the LV wall thickness by inclusion of accessory tendons and chords, papillary muscles, or trabeculae.
- Over-reporting a subaortic septal bulge in hypertensive patients, and the elderly as HCM.
- Overdiagnosis and reporting of moderate to severe concentric LVH as HCM without excluding other potential causes (Table 7.6).
- Overdiagnosing and reporting HCM in all patients with SAM and LVOTO.
- Misdiagnosis of apical HCM as acute coronary syndrome when apical wall endocardium is poorly visualised and may appear akinetic. Transpulmonary contrast will help confirm the diagnosis.
- Failing to search for LV apical aneurysm in patients with apical HCM and mid-cavity obstruction. Modified views, such as: very low LV parasternal short-axis (fourth to fifth left intercostal space) and laterally displaced apical 4-chamber and 3-chamber views (at posterior axillary line) may help identify very distal LV apical aneurysms.
- Missing a subaortic membrane as a cause of non-valve LV outflow acceleration and LV hypertrophy.
- Mistaking mitral regurgitation for the LV outflow jet on continuous-wave Doppler.
- Failing to perform provocation manoeuvres to uncover dynamic SAM, LVOTO, and mitral regurgitation.
- Failure to recognise and report specific features of conditions that mimic HCM (Table 7.10).

Restrictive Cardiomyopathy

- In a patient suspected of heart failure with no obvious LV hypertrophy or dilatation, restrictive cardiomyopathy is defined by:
  - Restrictive LV filling (mitral deceleration time <140 ms, mitral E/A >2.5, average E/E' >14)[4].
  - Normal or mildly reduced LV systolic function.
  - The causes are given in Table 7.11. An important differential diagnosis is pericardial constriction (see page 197).

Table 7.11 **Common restrictive cardiomyopathies**[13]

	Examples
Infiltrative	Amyloidosis (Table 7.10), sarcoidosis
Storage disease	Fabry (Table 7.10), Pompe, mucopolysaccharidosis
	Haemochromatosis (endocardial hyperechogenicity)
Non-infiltrative	Idiopathic, scleroderma, inherited myopathies
Endomyocardial	Endomyocardial fibrosis (Table 7.12)
Cancer therapy	Cancer and cancer therapies (e.g. anthracycline)

Table 7.12 **TTE features of endomyocardial fibrosis**

Echogenicity at RV or LV apex (Figure 7.2)
Sub-valve LV or RV thickening
LV or RV thrombus
Tricuspid or mitral regurgitation

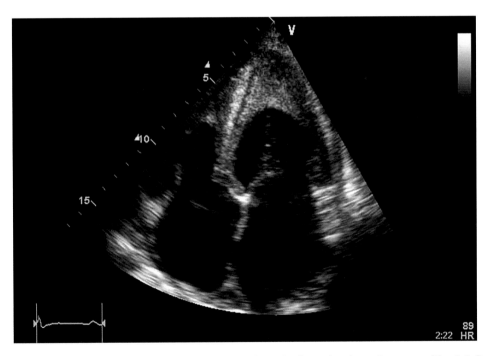

Figure 7.2 **Endomyocardial fibrosis.** There is thrombosis at the apex of both left and right ventricle.

And here's an electronic link to a loop on the website or use
http://goo.gl/hA9Ueh

Other imaging modalities:

- **CMR** is used for the detection of amyloidosis and haemochromatosis and **99mTc-DPD scintigraphy** for amyloidosis.

 MISTAKES TO AVOID

- Mistaking the presence of restrictive physiology for restrictive cardiomyopathy. Restrictive physiology occurs in any situation with a high filling pressure and rapid cessation of flow (e.g. post–myocardial infarction, pericardial constriction).

Non-Compaction

- The fetal heart is heavily trabeculated but becomes compacted during development. Non-compaction arises either from interruption of this process or the new growth of trabeculations later in life.
- New trabeculation can occur in other cardiomyopathies (dilated or hypertrophic) or physiological stimuli (e.g. exercise training).
- The presentation is classically with heart failure, ventricular arrhythmia, or systemic emboli, but the diagnosis may be made on family screening.
- The TTE shows numerous (>3), prominent trabeculations (Figure 7.3) (Table 7.13). Look for thrombus in the recesses.
- Assess LV size and function. Systolic function is often reduced initially at the area of hypertrabeculation.
- Other congenital cardiac abnormalities are commonly associated with non-compaction (e.g. ASD, VSD, transposition, tetralogy of Fallot).

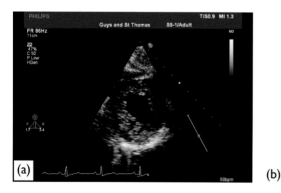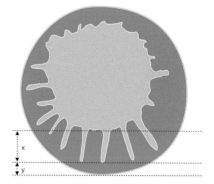

Figure 7.3 Non-compaction. (a) Parasternal short-axis view showing posterior trabeculation, and this is illustrated diagrammatically in (b). A ratio of non-compacted: compacted wall >2 (x/y) at end-systole is the commonly used Jenni diagnostic criterion[15].

Table 7.13 **Features of isolated ventricular non-compaction**[14]

>3 large trabeculae (usually at apex, mid-inferior, or lateral wall), with deep intertrabecular recesses (confirmed on colour mapping)
Ratio of non-compacted:compacted myocardium >2 on an end-systolic parasternal short-axis view[14] (Figure 7.3)
Absence of congenital causes of pressure load (e.g. LV outflow obstruction)
Associated features
Hypokinesis of affected segments
Dilatation and hypokinesis of unaffected segments, usually at the base of the LV
Abnormal ECG (LBBB, poor R wave progression, pathological Q waves)

- The differential diagnosis for hypertrabeculation[15] is:
  - Normal trabeculation in Afro-Caribbean people.
  - Trabeculation associated with athletic training, especially in Afro-Caribbean people.
  - Trabeculation in hypertrophic cardiomyopathy.
  - Trabeculation in dilated or peripartum cardiomyopathy.
  - False tendons.

Other imaging modalities:
- **CMR** may be useful, especially if TTE image quality is suboptimal. The diagnosis is suggested by a non-compacted:compacted ratio >2.3 at end-diastole.

Arrhythmogenic Right Ventricle Cardiomyopathy/Dysplasia (ARVC/ARVD)

- The diagnosis is based on a combination of histology, imaging (echo and magnetic resonance), ECG, arrhythmias, and family history.
- TTE is part of the initial evaluation of a patient with suspected ARVC and for follow-up at one- to two-year intervals, based on age, genetic status, and clinical features.
- TTE changes include RV dilatation, reduced RV systolic function, and regional wall motion abnormalities, such as akinesis, dyskinesis, or aneurysms (Figures 4.1 and 7.4) (Table 7.14).
- The most commonly affected regions of the RV are the infundibulum, apex, inferolateral wall, and peri-tricuspid annulus[16].

- LV involvement is common and may sometimes dominate with:
  - Non-dilated and globally hypokinetic LV.
  - Regional wall motion abnormalities often starting inferolaterally.
- Other causes of RV dilatation and dysfunction that should be considered are:
  - RV infarct.
  - Dilated cardiomyopathy confined to the RV.
  - Pulmonary artery hypertension.

Table 7.14 **Echocardiographic features of arrhythmogenic RV cardiomyopathy/dysplasia**[17, 18]*

Major criteria	
PLAX RVOT	≥32 mm (≥19 mm/m²)
PSAX RVOT	≥36 mm (≥21 mm/m²)
RV fractional area change**	≤33%
Minor criteria	
PLAX RVOT	≥29 mm to <32 mm (≥16 ≤18 mm/m²)
PSAX RVOT	≥32 mm to <36 mm (≥18 ≤20 mm/m²)
RV fractional area change**	>33% to ≤40%

* Regional RV akinesia, dyskinesia, or aneurysm and RV dilatation shown by one of the following (end-diastole).

** Measured by tracing the RV endocardium in systole and diastole in the 4-chamber view. Subtract the systolic area from the diastolic area and divide by the diastolic area, then multiply by 100.

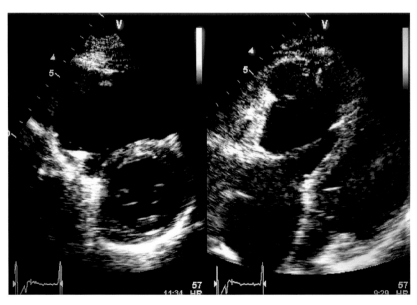

Figure 7.4 **ARVC/D.** On the left is a short-axis view, and on the right, a modified RV apical view, showing a markedly dilated RV with aneurysms.

- Congenital heart diseases, for example, ASD, Ebstein's anomaly.
- Severe pectus excavatum.

Other imaging modalities:
- **CMR** is the most accurate imaging modality for the detection of early ARVC[16].
- The peri-tricuspid area and the LV inferolateral wall may be the only affected regions[16].

Cardio-Oncology: Evaluation of Patients on Chemotherapy

- Echocardiography is used for the evaluation of patients in preparation for, during, and after cancer therapy.
- **Choice of TTE protocol:**
  - Baseline imaging requires a comprehensive TTE.
  - A focused study may be sufficient for surveillance during potentially cardiotoxic cancer treatments (internally agreed with oncology team).

1. LV and RV systolic and diastolic function
- Accurate and reproducible assessment of LV systolic function is critical for patients exposed to potentially cardiotoxic chemotherapeutic agents[2, 4].
- A cut point <53% is used for a reduced LV ejection fraction in cardio-oncology protocols[2, 4]. However, in practice it is nearly impossible to provide this level of accuracy.
- **Recommended methods for the assessment of LV systolic function:**
  - **3D volume–derived LV ejection fraction and 2D GLS** (FR 50–80 Hz) when images are of good quality. Ideally, use vendor-neutral software for all 3D data analysis. Otherwise, use the same dedicated system for serial studies, and strongly consider a single operator.
  - For 3D data analysis, use multibeat acquisition (4–6 cycles) and frame rates >20 Hz.
  - **2D Simpson's biplane LV ejection fraction and 2D GLS**. If GLS is not possible, use TDI S' lateral.
- **Have a low threshold for using a contrast agent** if images are of suboptimal quality.
- LV diastolic function and RV dysfunction have not been found to be prognostic of cardiotoxicity.
- Immediately report any of the following to the cardio-oncology team[18] (Figure 7.5):

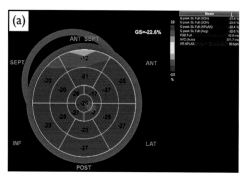 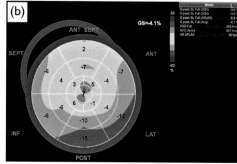

Figure 7.5 **Role of GLS in cardio-oncology.** (a) Bull's-eye representation of GLS in a normal LV; (b) Bull's-eye representation of an impaired LV with significantly reduced GLS in a patient having Herceptin.

Table 7.15 **Frequency of TTE according to chemotherapeutic agent**[2, 4, 19]

Toxicity type	Drugs examples	Measurements	F/U TTE
Type I *Permanent damage Cumulative dose Risk of heart failure and death*	Doxorubicin Epirubicin Idarubicin	LVEF >53% GLS <–16% Troponin negative	End of treatment and six months later
		LVEF <53% GLS >–16% Troponin positive	Guided by cardiology review
Type II *Reversible effects Not dose-related No apparent structural damage*	Trastuzumab Lapatinib Pertuzumab	LVEF >53% GLS <–16% Troponin negative	Every three months during treatment
		LVEF <53% GLS >–16% Troponin positive	Guided by cardiology review

- **10% reduction in serial LV ejection fraction** to below the lower limit of normal (50–55%).
- **15% reduction in GLS**.
- **GLS of >–16% (absolute value <16%)** regardless of interval change.
- Guideline frequencies for serial TTE are given in Table 7.15.

2. Look at the valves and pericardium
- Heart valve disease may precede the cancer or may arise as a result of radiotherapy, LV dysfunction, or infective or thrombotic non-infective endocarditis.
- Patients with baseline or changing valve abnormalities should have serial TTE during and after treatment[4].

● Pericardial disease may be secondary to cardiac metastases or a consequence of radiotherapy or chemotherapy (see Chapter 17).

CHECKLIST REPORT IN CARDIOMYOPATHY

1. LV dimensions, wall thickness (location of any hypertrophy), and morphology, including trabeculation.
2. LV regional and global systolic and diastolic function.
3. LV thrombus?
4. In suspected HCM—systolic anterior motion of the mitral valve with secondary LVOT acceleration +/– mitral regurgitation (including changes with Valsalva and standing).
5. In suspected HCM—echocardiographic risk factors for sudden death: wall thickness ≥30 mm, LA >48 mm, LA volume >34 mL/m^2, LV ejection fraction <50%, LVOT obstruction >50 mmHg.
6. RV size and function. RVOT dilatation in ARVC.
7. Pulmonary pressure.
8. Valve function as a cause of LV dilatation, but also secondary mitral regurgitation as a complication.

References

1. Elliott P, Andersson B, Arbustini E, et. al. Classification of the cardiomyopathies: A position statement from the European Society of Cardiology Working Group on Myocardial and Pericardial Diseases. Eur Heart J 2008;29(2):270–76.
2. Merlo M, Cannatà A, Gobbo M, Stolfo D, Elliott PM & Sinagra G. Evolving concepts in dilated cardiomyopathy. Europ J Heart Failure 2018;20(2):228–39.
3. Pinto YM, Elliott PM, Arbustini E, et al. Proposal for a revised definition of dilated cardiomyopathy, hypokinetic non-dilated cardiomyopathy, and its implications for clinical practice: A position statement of the ESC Working Group on Myocardial and Pericardial Diseases. Eur Heart J 2016;37(23):1850–58.
4. Plana JC, Galderisi M, Barac A, et al. Expert consensus for multimodality imaging evaluation of adult patients during and after cancer therapy: A report from the American Society of Echocardiography and the European Association of Cardiovascular Imaging. Europ Heart J 2014;15:1063–93.
5. Galderisi M, Cardim N, D'Andrea A, et al. The multi-modality cardiac imaging approach to the athlete's heart: An expert consensus of the European Association of Cardiovascular Imaging. Europ Heart J CVI 2015;16(4):353a–t.
6. Richand V, Lafitte S, Reant P, et al. An ultrasound speckle tracking (two-dimensional strain) analysis of myocardial deformation in professional soccer players compared with healthy subjects and hypertrophic cardiomyopathy. Am J Cardiol 2007;100(1):128–32.

7. Houston B & Mukherjee M. Cardiac sarcoidosis: Clinical manifestations, imaging characteristics, and therapeutic approach. Clin Med Insights in Cardiol 2014;8(Suppl 1):31–7.

8. Marques. JS & Pinto FJ. Clinical use of multimodality imaging in the assessment of dilated cardiomyopathy. Heart on Line 2015;101(7):565–72.

9. Elliott PM, Anastasakis A, Borger MA, et al. 2014 ESC Guidelines on diagnosis and management of hypertrophic cardiomyopathy. Europ Heart J 2014;35(39):2733–79.

10. Turvey L, Augustine DX, Robinson S, et al. Transthoracic echocardiography of hypertrophic cardiomyopathy in adults: A practical guideline from the British Society of Echocardiography. Echo Research and Practice 2021;8(1):G61–86.

11. Rowin EJ, Maron BJ, Haas TS, et al. Hypertrophic cardiomyopathy with left ventricular apical aneurysm: Implications for risk stratification and management. J Am Coll Cardiol 2017;69(7):761–73.

12. Hiemstra YL, Debonnaire P, Bootsma M, et al. Global longitudinal strain and left atrial volume index provide incremental prognostic value in patients with hypertrophic cardiomyopathy. Circulation: CVI 2017;10(7):e005706.

13. Muchtar E, Blauwet LA & Gertz MA. Restrictive cardiomyopathy genetics, pathogenesis, clinical manifestations, diagnosis, and therapy. Circ Res 2017;121(7):819–37.

14. Jenni R, Oechslin E, Schneider J, Attenhofer JC & Kaufmann PA. Echocardiographic and pathoanatomical characteristics of isolated left ventricular non-compaction: A step towards classification as a distinct cardiomyopathy. Heart 2001;86(6):666–71.

15. Nagueh SF, Smiseth AO, Appleton CP, et al. ASE/EACVI Guidelines and standards. Recommendations for the evaluation of left ventricular diastolic function by echocardiography: An update from the American Society of Echocardiography and the European Association of Cardiovascular Imaging. J Am Soc Echocardiogr 2016;29(4):277–314.

16. Corrado D, Van Tintelen PJ, J. McKenna WJ, et al. Arrhythmogenic right ventricular cardiomyopathy: Evaluation of the current diagnostic criteria and differential diagnosis. Europ Heart J 2020;41(14):1414–27.

17. Marcus FI, McKenna WJ, Sherill D, et al. Diagnosis of arrhythmogenic right ventricular cardiomyopathy/dysplasia. Proposed modifications of the task force criteria. Circulation 2010;121(13):1533–41.

18. Towbin JA, McKenna WJ, Abrams DJ, et al. HRS expert consensus statement on evaluation, risk stratification, and management of arrhythmogenic cardiomyopathy. Heart Rhythm 2019;16(11):e301–72.

19. Dobson R, Ghosh AK, Ky B, et al. British Society for Echocardiography and British Cardio-Oncology Society guideline for transthoracic echocardiographic assessment of adult cancer patients receiving anthracyclines and/or trastuzumab. Echo Research and Practice 2021;8(1):G1–8.

Aortic Valve Disease

8

Aortic Stenosis

1. Appearance of the valve and aorta

- Describe the valve in detail. Look at the number of cusps, pattern of thickening, and mobility on zoomed views. These may give a clue to the aetiology (Table 8.1).
- A bicuspid aortic valve may only be obvious in systole (Figure 8.1).
- If the valve is bicuspid:
  - Is it anatomical or functional (two cusps fused either partially or fully with a median raphe).
  - Which cusps are fused? Fusion of right and left cusps is the most common pattern and more likely to be associated with aortic dilatation and coarctation[1].
  - Is the valve thickened and restricted or thin and normally functioning? More than mild thickening and restriction predicts faster progression to surgery[2].
- Assess the aorta at all levels (see page 161).
- With a bicuspid aortic valve, the sinus, sinotubular junction, or ascending aorta may be dilated.
- If the ascending aorta cannot be imaged adequately even after moving the probe a space higher than for the parasternal views or in a right intercostal space, consider CMR or CT scanning.

Table 8.1 **Clues to the aetiology in aortic stenosis**

	Systolic bowing	Closure line	Associated features
Calcific disease	No	Central	Calcification of mitral annulus or aorta
Bicuspid	Yes	Often eccentric	Ascending aortic dilatation, coarctation
Rheumatic	Yes	Central	Mitral involvement

DOI: 10.1201/9781003242789-8

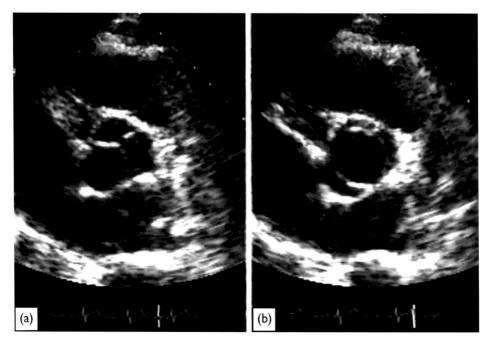

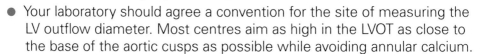

Figure 8.1 **Bicuspid aortic valve in systole and diastole.** In diastole, (a) the valve may look tricuspid if there is only mild fusion and no raphe. Only in systole (b) with the valve open will it be obvious that two cusps are partly fused. The fusion may affect only a small length of the cusp edge adjacent to the commissure.

- The aorta may be replaced at a diameter of 45 mm if aortic valve surgery is independently indicated[3, 4].
- About 5% of bicuspid valves are associated with coarctation.

2. Doppler measurements

- The minimum dataset[5] is V_{max}, mean gradient and effective orifice area using the continuity equation (Figure 8.2).

- Your laboratory should agree a convention for the site of measuring the LV outflow diameter. Most centres aim as high in the LVOT as close to the base of the aortic cusps as possible while avoiding annular calcium.
- Check that the measured LVOT diameter is the same as last time. If not, we suggest:
  - Use the better of the two measurements (taking into account image quality and measurement technique).
  - In your summary, report the EOA, calculated using the optimal diameter for your own and the previous study for consistency.
  - This is particularly important if you are measuring the diameter at the base of the aortic cusps when previously a point was taken within the cylindrical part of the LVOT.

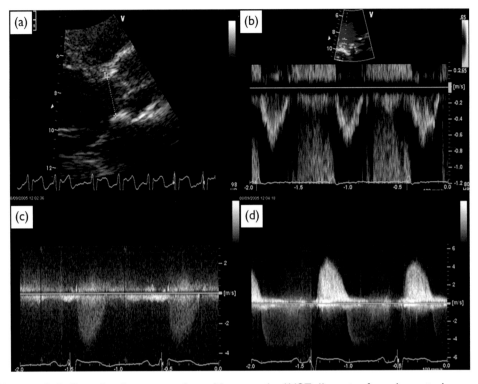

Figure 8.2 **Continuity equation.** Measure the LVOT diameter from inner to inner edge (a) as high as possible towards the base of the cusps avoiding annular calcification. (b) Record the pulsed signal in the centre of the LVOT as flow accelerates, moving the pulsed sample up and down until a stable signal is obtained. Record the continuous wave signal using a stand-alone probe from the apex (c) and right intercostal space (d) and use the optimal signal, in this case (d). Trace the modal or dense part of the signal, avoiding artefact.

- Record the continuous waveform using the stand-alone probe from the apex and at least one other approach (usually suprasternal or right intercostal), unless the aortic valve disease is obviously mild, shown by all of:
  - Mobile cusps
  - V_{max} <3.0 m/s
  - Normal LV ejection fraction

3. **Assess severity**
   - If the aortic valve is thickened with a V_{max} <2.5 m/s and normal LV ejection fraction, report 'aortic valve thickening with no stenosis'.
   - If the V_{max} ≥2.5 m/s, grade as in Table 8.2 if all measurements agree. If there is disagreement, see Section 3.1 or 3.2.

Table 8.2 **Severity in aortic stenosis: Main criteria**[5]

	Mild	Moderate	Severe
Transaortic V_{max} (m/s)	2.6–2.9	3.0–4.0	>4.0
Peak gradient (mmHg)	<40	40–65	>65
Mean gradient (mmHg)	<20	20–40	>40
EOA (continuity equation) (cm²)	>1.5	1.0–1.5	<1.0

Table 8.3 **Severity in aortic stenosis: Extra criteria**

	Mild	Moderate	Severe
Waveform shape (Figure 8.3)	Dagger	Dagger	Arch
Indexed EOA (cm²/m²)	>0.85	0.60–0.85	<0.60
Dimensionless index	>0.50	0.25–0.50	<0.25

3.1 If the V_{max} suggests severe (>4.0 m/s) but the EOA suggests only moderate (>1.0 cm²)

This arises because of:

- High flow (aortic regurgitation, anaemia, anxiety)
- Errors of measurement

You need to:

- **Check your measurements**. Was the pulsed sample too close to the valve? Check the LV outflow diameter against previous measurements.
- **Consider the dimensionless index** (Table 8.3). If the LV outflow diameter is unreliably large, the dimensionless index gives a guide to severity. It should be calculated as $VTI_{subaortic}/VTI_{av}$. Do not use the ratio of subaortic to aortic V_{max}.
- **Look again at the valve appearance**. Is the valve calcified and immobile, suggesting severe AS, or are the tips mobile, suggesting more moderate AS?
- **Look at the waveform shape**[5] (Figure 8.3 and Table 8.3). A dagger shape suggests moderate stenosis, and an arch shape suggests severe stenosis.
- **Correct for body surface area** (Table 8.3). Correction for BSA should not be done routinely, because it will tend to categorise too many people as having severe aortic stenosis, but it is helpful in uncertain cases. If the patient is large, a corrected EOA may be in the severe range despite a moderate uncorrected EOA (Box 8.1).

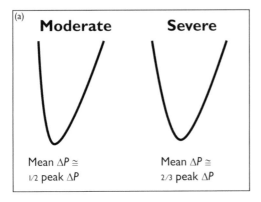
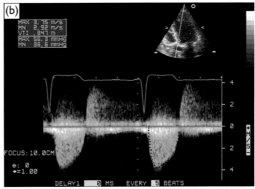
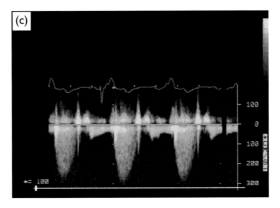

Figure 8.3 **Continuous waveform shape.** (a) Left panel. In moderate aortic stenosis, the upstroke is relatively quick, giving a dagger-shaped signal in which the mean gradient is approximately half the peak. Right panel. In severe stenosis, the ejection time lengthens and the acceleration time to peak velocity also lengthens. This causes an arch shape in which the mean gradient is approximately 2/3 the peak gradient. (b) shows a waveform in moderate disease, and (c) a waveform in severe disease.

Box 8.1 Correcting effective orifice area for body surface area (BSA)

Assuming an EOA 1.3 cm²:

- If the patient is 6 ft tall and weighs 120 kg, the BSA is 2.4 m², giving EOAi 0.54 cm²/m², indicating severe AS.
- If the patient is 5 ft tall and weighs 50 kg, the BSA is 1.45 m² and the EOAi is 0.9 cm²/m², indicating mild AS.

3.2 If the V_{max} suggests moderate (<4.0 m/s), but the EOA suggests severe (<1.0 cm²)

This can be for a number of reasons:

- The cut points between the grades are, to a degree, arbitrary, and an EOA 0.8–1.0 cm² may be moderate, especially in smaller people[6] (Box 8.1).
- Low flow causes a fall in V_{max} despite severe aortic stenosis.
- Errors of measurement.

You need to:

- **Check your measurements**. The likeliest errors are in placing the pulsed sample too far towards the LV apex and in underestimating LVOT diameter (check the value found in previous studies).
- **Look again at the valve appearance**. Is the valve calcified and fixed, suggesting severe AS, or are the tips mobile, suggesting moderate AS?
- **Look at the waveform shape**[5] (Figure 8.4 and Table 8.3). A dagger shape suggests moderate stenosis, and an arch shape suggests severe.
- **Correct for body surface area if the patient is small.**
- **Consider measuring the area of the LV outflow tract on 3D** since it may not be circular and may be underestimated from the linear diameter.
- **Consider low-gradient, low-flow AS** (see 3.3).

3.3 Low-gradient, low-flow aortic stenosis

This occurs if:

- The LV ejection fraction is low, usually <50% ('classical low-flow, low-gradient AS').
  - The low LV ejection fraction is likely caused solely by the AS and, unless very low, will improve after intervention.

- The LV cavity is small despite a normal ejection fraction >50% ('paradoxical low-flow, low-gradient AS'). Even with a normal or high LV ejection fraction, the volume of blood ejected is small.
  - There may be LV disease (e.g. from hypertension, or amyloid) separate from the AS, and the differentiation of these can be difficult and require further tests.
  - Conventionally, a stroke volume index <35 mL/m² is used to define this entity, although this is not a measure of flow.
  - Occasionally, true flow, calculated as (stroke volume)/(systolic ejection time), may be low despite a normal stroke volume index. A flow < 200 mL/s is usually taken as low.
- Or there is severe mitral stenosis or regurgitation or a VSD.

4. **If the diagnosis is not clear, discuss the case to consider further action:**

4.1 Consider low-dose dobutamine stress echocardiography

- This is indicated for a V_{max} <3.5 m/s with an LV ejection fraction <40%.
- It is not usually indicated if:
  - The V_{max} is >3.5 m/s, especially if the LV ejection fraction is <40%, since this is almost certainly severe aortic stenosis[7].
  - The LV cavity is small and the LV ejection fraction is normal, since severe LV outflow acceleration may occur, making accurate measurement impossible and risking cardiac arrhythmia.

- It requires medical supervision because of the risk of cardiac arrhythmia:
  - Give 5 then 10 μg/kg/min dobutamine (occasionally 20 μg/kg/min, especially if prior beta blockade).
  - Stop the infusion if the $VTI_{subaortic}$ rises >20% or the heart rate increases.
  - Judge the severity of AS and whether there is LV contractile reserve (Table 8.4). If the $VTI_{subaortic}$ fails to rise by >20%, consider calculating the change in flow (see 3.3 or Appendix for calculation).
  - In the absence of contractile reserve, the risk at aortic valve replacement is high[8].

Table 8.4 **Stress echocardiography in low-flow aortic stenosis**[8]

Is there severe aortic stenosis?
Mean gradient >40 mmHg and EOA <1.0 cm² at any time during stress
Is there LV contractile reserve?
Subaortic velocity time integral (or ejection fraction or flow) rises by >20%

4.2 Consider CT calcium scoring

This is useful in 'paradoxical low-flow, low-gradient AS' when the valve is calcified and the LV ejection fraction is normal.

4.3 Clinical correlates

A review of the case correlating clinical characteristics, imaging, and biomarkers is often needed (Table 8.5), unless the grade is clear.

5. **General**
- Assess aortic regurgitation (page 90).
- Assess the aorta.

Table 8.5 Differentiating moderate and severe aortic stenosis with mean gradient <40 mmHg and EOA <1.0 cm² and EF >50%[4]

	Likely moderate	Likely severe
EOA (cm²)	0.8–1.0	<0.8
V_{max} (m/s)	<3.5	3.5–3.9
Continuous wave signal shape	Dagger	Arch
Valve appearance	Cusp tips still open	Heavily calcified and immobile
Patient characteristics	Small and asymptomatic	Symptoms
SVi (mL/m²)	>35	<35
CT calcium score (A units)	<1,600 for men, <800 for women	>2,000 for men, >1,200 for women

- If the ascending aorta cannot be imaged by TTE, a CT scan or CMR should be requested. These can also assess the whole of the rest of the aorta.
- If there is apparent heavy aortic calcification, then a CT scan is indicated to look for a 'porcelain aorta', which may contraindicate surgical valve replacement.

● Assess the other valves. Secondary (functional) mitral regurgitation may develop in severe aortic stenosis if the LV is dilated. Mitral surgery is likely to be necessary if:
- The mitral valve is anatomically abnormal (e.g. prolapsing).
- The secondary mitral regurgitation is moderate to severe or severe.

● Estimate pulmonary artery pressure (see Chapter 5).
- Pulmonary hypertension is no longer included as an indication for intervention in asymptomatic severe AS.
- However, pulmonary hypertension is common (usually taken as a PA systolic pressure >60 mmHg) and carries a poor prognosis without aortic valve intervention[9].
- A rise in tricuspid regurgitation V_{max} from the last study alerts to a change and may be used to help decide the need for intervention if other measures are equivocal.

● Note LV outflow hypertrophy, which has a number of possible consequences:
- It may contribute to high flow velocities across the aortic valve.
- It may affect a TAVI procedure (see 7).

- If severe, it increases risk at surgery.
- Post-operatively, it can cause HCM-like physiology with low cardiac output, especially with excessive inotropes and diuretic therapy.

- If there is a discrepancy in the pressure difference and the appearance of the valve, check for a subaortic membrane.

6. Is surgery indicated on TTE?[4, 5]

Aortic valve surgery is most clearly indicated for severe AS and symptoms. However, in asymptomatic patients or patients having CABG, the TTE can aid the decision for surgery (Table 8.6).

Table 8.6 **Echocardiographic and other indications for surgery in asymptomatic aortic stenosis**[3, 4]

Echocardiographic indications	Class
Moderate or severe AS having CABG or aortic replacement	I
Severe AS and LV ejection fraction <50% with no other cause	I
Severe AS and LV ejection fraction <55%[4] or a progressive decrease to <60% on three successive studies[3]	2a 2b
Transaortic V_{max} >5.0 m/s or EOA <0.6 cm²	2a
Severe coexistent aortic dilatation (see page 165)	I
Increase in V_{max} ≥0.3 m/s in one year associated with severe calcification[4]	2a
Non-echocardiographic indications	
Symptoms on exercise test	I
Fall in BP >20 mmHg on exercise	2a
B-type natriuretic peptide level raised by >3 times normal[4]	2a

7. Transcatheter valve (TAVI) workup (Table 8.7)

- Measure the echocardiographic 'annulus' taken from inner to inner edge at the base of the cusps[10]. This is needed for sizing the valve.
- The annulus may be oval. Further assessment of the annulus size and shape may be performed at the TAVI centre using 3D TOE at the time of the procedure or beforehand if there is significant uncertainty[11].
- CT is routine for assessing: the annulus (area, perimeter, diameters, shape, and calcification), the height of the coronary ostia above the annulus, the whole thoracic aorta and peripheral arteries.

Table 8.7 Echocardiographic features in the TAVI workup

Aorta	
Heavy calcification	Confirms TAVI more suitable than surgical replacement
Annulus diameter	Used for sizing
Diameter at sinus and STJ	Dilatation (>45 mm) may contraindicate CoreValve
Left ventricle	
LV cavity size	If small, contraindicates transapical approach
Severe subaortic bulge	May contraindicate SAPIEN
Valves	
Bicuspid valve	Caution with some types of device
Heavy calcification of left cusp	Caution re-occlusion of left main stem during the procedure
Severe mitral regurgitation	May favour conventional surgery

Abbreviation: STJ is sinotubular junction.

 # MISTAKES TO AVOID

- Mistaking the continuous wave signal from an eccentric jet of mitral regurgitation for aortic stenosis.
- Failing to recognise severe aortic stenosis if the V_{max} or mean gradient is in the moderate range but the EOA is low.
- Underestimating the degree of aortic stenosis by not using a stand-alone probe from at least two windows.
- Failing to detect dilatation of the ascending aorta, which is common if there is a bicuspid aortic valve.
- Missing a subaortic membrane. Recheck if the valve looks relatively mildly affected but the velocities are high.

Aortic Regurgitation

1. **Appearance of the valve and aorta**
   - Describe the valve in detail. Look at the number and mobility of the cusps on zoomed views (see Figure 8.1 for bicuspid aortic valve).

- Measure the aorta at every standard level (see page 161).
- This may allow you to determine the aetiology (Table 8.8).

2. Colour flow mapping

- Measure the jet height 5–10 mm below the cusps (on 2D or colour M-mode) (Figure 8.4) and express as a percentage of the diameter of the LVOT at the same level.
- If the jet is eccentric, the width must be taken perpendicular to its axis. If it is so eccentric that it impinges on the septum or anterior mitral leaflet, do not make the measurement.
- The width of the narrowest portion of the jet (the vena contracta) can also be used (Table 8.8) even if the jet is eccentric.

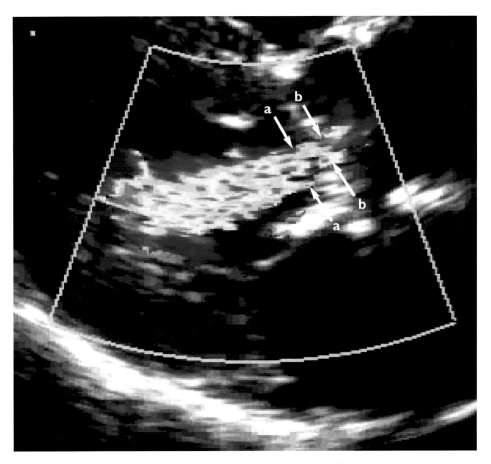

Figure 8.4 **Regurgitant jet.** Parasternal long-axis view. The position for measuring the height of the colour flow map as a percentage of the outflow tract height is at (a). The vena contracta or neck is at (b).

Table 8.8 **Aetiology of aortic regurgitation**

Dilatation of root or ascending aorta	
(Table 15.1)	
Valve	
Common	Bicuspid, rheumatic, calcific disease, endocarditis
Uncommon	Prolapse, irradiation, drugs,* antiphospholipid syndrome, carcinoid

* Cabergoline, pergolide, fenfluramine, benfluorex.

3. **Continuous wave signal**
   - Record either from the apex or, if the jet is directed posteriorly, from the parasternal position.
   - Measure the pressure half-time and note the density of the signal compared with the density of forward flow.

4. **Flow reversal at the arch**
   - From the suprasternal notch, describe:
     - Whether flow reversal is holodiastolic, fills approximately half of diastole, or is only seen at the start of diastole using colour M-mode (Figure 8.5) and pulsed Doppler (Figure 8.6).
     - How far down the aorta can flow reversal be detected on colour mapping.

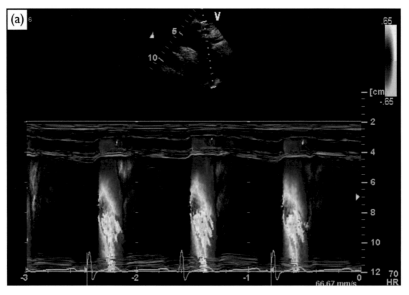

Figure 8.5 **Flow reversal on colour mapping in the upper descending thoracic aorta.** Using a suprasternal position colour M-mode in a patient with mild regurgitation (a) illustrates localised and short-lived flow reversal. In severe regurgitation, (b) flow reversal is holodiastolic across the whole aortic lumen and seen well down the descending thoracic aorta.

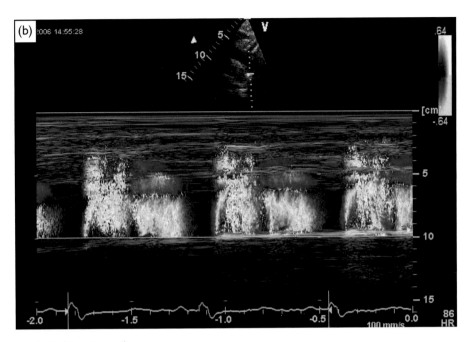

Figure 8.5 (Continued)

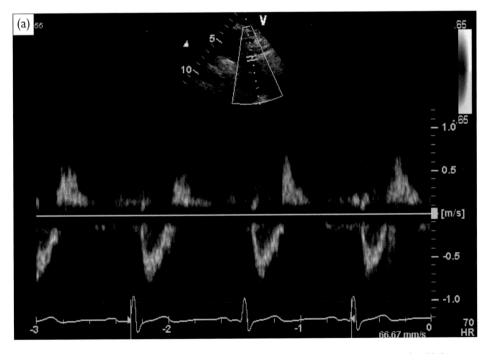

Figure 8.6 **Flow reversal on pulsed Doppler in the distal arch.** Using a suprasternal position, mild regurgitation causes (a) short-lived low-velocity reversal, while in severe regurgitation, (b) the reversal is holodiastolic, with a relatively high velocity at the end of diastole (e.g. ≥ 0.2 m/s)[12].

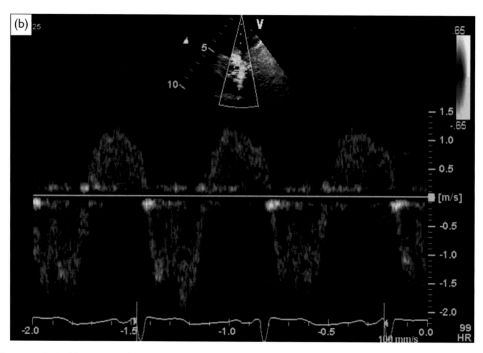

Figure 8.6 (Continued)

5. **Grade the severity of regurgitation**
   - Make an assessment based on all modalities. The height of the colour jet in the LVOT and flow reversal beyond the arch are the most reliable modalities (Table 8.9).
   - The PISA technique is not routinely used for aortic regurgitation.

Table 8.9 **Criteria of severity in aortic regurgitation**[13]

	Mild	Moderate	Severe
Colour/LVOT height (%)	<25	25–64	≥65
Vena contracta width (mm)	<3	3–6	>6
Flow reversal in descending aorta	None	Not holodiastolic	Holodiastolic
Pressure half-time (ms)	>500	200–500	<200*
CW signal intensity	Faint or incomplete waveform	Intermediate	Dense as forward flow

* The pressure half-time depends on LV diastolic pressure and systemic vascular resistance and may be short with LV dysfunction even if the aortic regurgitation is mild or moderate.

6. The left ventricle

- Is the LV hyperdynamic (suggesting severe aortic regurgitation)?
- Chronic severe regurgitation usually causes LV diastolic dilatation. In acute regurgitation, the LV diastolic volume may be normal.
- Measure LV volumes. The LV becomes more spherical in severe aortic regurgitation, and linear dimensions may then be unrepresentative of LV size. No guideline cut point for surgery exists, but a progressive increase in volume may still be clinically useful.
- LV TDI or GLS can corroborate a decline in other measures of LV function but cannot be used alone as indications for surgery.

7. Are there echocardiographic criteria for surgery?[3, 4]

See Table 8.10. In individual cases, two or more of these indications may summate.

Table 8.10 Echocardiographic and other indications for surgery in asymptomatic aortic regurgitation[3, 4]

Indications for surgery	Class
Moderate or severe AR having CABG or aortic replacement	I
Severe AR and LV ejection fraction ≤50%[4] or ≤55%[3] with no other cause	I
LV systolic diameter >50 mm or 25 mm/m^2	I[4] 2a[3]
Low-risk surgery, severe AR, and progressive fall in LV ejection fraction to <60% on ≥3 serial studies[3]	2b
Low risk for surgery and LV systolic diameter >20 mm/m^2 if the patient is small or LV ejection fraction ≤55%[4]	2b
Progressive increase in LV diastolic diameter to >65 mm[3, 4] or fall in LV ejection fraction to <60% on ≥3 serial studies[3]	2b
Severe coexistent aortic dilatation (see page 165)	I

8. Assess the other valves and right heart

- Mitral regurgitation may occur secondary to LV dilatation.
- Pulmonary hypertension is much less common than in severe aortic stenosis.

Other techniques in aortic stenosis and regurgitation

- **CMR**
  - Shows valve morphology if TTE windows are suboptimal.
  - Shows the rest of the aorta if only the root can be imaged adequately on TTE.

- Estimates the regurgitant fraction if the grade of regurgitation is uncertain on TTE.
- Calculates LV volume and function if image quality is suboptimal on TTE.

- **CT**
  - Shows the whole aorta for dimensions and the presence of excess calcification.
  - Images coronary arteries in selected patients before valve intervention.
  - TAVI workup (see Table 8.7).

Acute Aortic Regurgitation

This is caused mainly by infective endocarditis. The LV and general circulation have not had time to adapt, and the LV may be hyperdynamic but not yet dilated. The risk of decompensation and death is high:

- Measure transmitral E deceleration time (Figure 8.7).
- Use continuous wave Doppler across the mitral valve to look for diastolic mitral regurgitation (Figure 8.7). This is a sign of immediate LV decompensation and an indication for emergency surgery[15].
- Inform the clinician in charge of the case immediately if the E deceleration time is <150 ms or if there is diastolic mitral regurgitation.

MISTAKES TO AVOID

- Placing the pulsed sample in the distal arch too close to the aortic wall. This produces signal artefacts late in diastole (signal symmetrical above and below the baseline), which can be mistaken for flow reversal.
- Missing a transmitral deceleration time <150 ms as a sign of imminent decompensation in acute aortic regurgitation.
- Overestimating AR using AR pressure half-time shortened by a high LVEDP as a result of coexistent LV disease.
- Using vena contracta cut points to assess the jet width in the LVOT.
- Measuring pressure half-time when not fully aligned to the regurgitant jet. The AR jet initial peak velocity is usually about 4 m/s with a normal blood pressure. If much lower, especially with a bidirectional signal, use other methods to evaluate the degree of regurgitation.

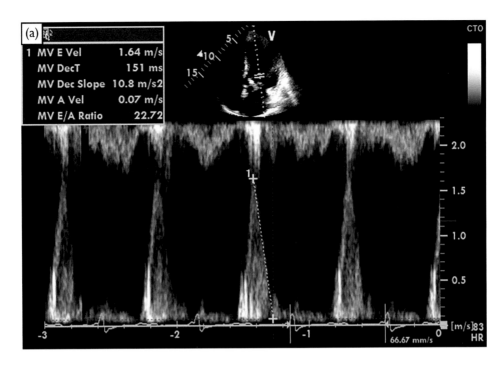

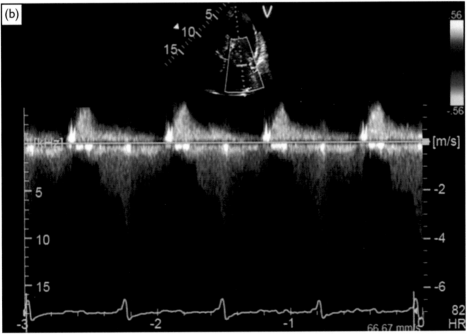

Figure 8.7 **Spectral Doppler signals in acute aortic regurgitation.** These signals were recorded soon before decompensation and death in a patient with acute severe aortic regurgitation caused by endocarditis. In (a), the E deceleration time is shortened to 151 ms, and in (b), there is prolonged diastolic mitral regurgitation.

CHECKLIST REPORT IN AORTIC VALVE DISEASE

1. Appearance and movement of the aortic valve.
2. Grade of stenosis and regurgitation.
3. Size of aorta and check for coarctation.
4. LV dimensions and systolic function.
5. RV size and function and PA pressure (for aortic stenosis).
6. Other valves, particularly the mitral valve.

References

1. Schaefer BM, Lewin MB, Stout KK, Gill E, Prueitt A, Byers PH & Otto CM. The bicuspid aortic valve: An integrated phenotypic classification of leaflet morphology and aortic root shape. Heart 2008;94(12):1634–8.
2. Michelena HI, Desjardins VA, Avierinos JF, et al. Natural history of asymptomatic patients with normally functioning or minimally dysfunctional bicuspid aortic valve in the community. Circulation 2008;117(21):2776–84.
3. Otto CM, Nishimura RA, Bonow RO, et al. 2020 ACC/AHA Guideline for the management of patients with valvular heart disease: A report of the American College of Cardiology/American Heart Association Joint Committee on Clinical Practice Guidelines. Circulation 2021;143(5):e72–227.
4. Vahanian A, Beyersdorf F, Praz F, et al. 2021 ESC/EACTS Guidelines for the management of valvular heart disease. Eur Heart J 2022;43(7):561–632.
5. Baumgartner H, Hung J, Bermejo J, et al. Recommendations on the echocardiographic assessment of aortic valve stenosis: A focused update from the European Association of Cardiovascular Imaging and the American Society of Echocardiography. Europ Heart J CVI 2017;18(3):254–75.
6. Minners J, Allgeir M, Gohlke-Baerwolf C, Kienzle RP, Neuman FJ & Jander N. Inconsistencies of echocardiographic criteria for the grading of aortic stenosis. Europ Heart J 2008;29(8):1043–8.
7. Kellermair J, Saeed S, Chambers J, Kammler J, Blessberger H, Kiblboeck D, Grund M, Lambert T & Steinwender C. Predictors of true-severe classical low-flow low-gradient aortic stenosis at resting echocardiography. Int J Cardiol 2021;335:93–7.
8. Monin J-L, Quere J-P, Moncho M, et al. Low-gradient aortic stenosis. Operative risk stratification and predictors for long-term outcome: A multicenter study using dobutamine stress hemodynamics. Circulation 2003;108(3):319–24.
9. Cam A, Goel SS, Agarwal S, Menon V, Svensson LG, Tuzcu EM & Kapadia SR. Prognostic implications of pulmonary hypertension in patients with severe aortic stenosis. J Thorac Cardiovasc Surg 2011;142(8):800–8.

10. Zamorano JL, Badano LP, Bruce C, et al. EAE/ASE Recommendations for the use of echocardiography in new transcatheter interventions for valvular heart disease. Europ Heart J 2011;32(17):2189–4.
11. Rajani R, Hancock J & Chambers J. Imaging: The art of TAVI. Heart 2012;98 (Suppl 4):iv14–22.
12. Tribouilloy C, Avinee P, Shen WF, et al. End-diastolic flow velocity just beneath the aortic isthmus assessed by pulsed Doppler echocardiography: A new predictor of the aortic regurgitant fraction. Brit Heart J 1991;65(1):37–40.
13. Lancellotti P, Tribouilloy C, Hagendorff A, et al. European Association of Echocardiography recommendations for the assessment of valvular regurgitation. Part 1: Aortic and pulmonary regurgitation (native valve disease). Europ J Echo 2010;11(3):223–44.
14. Detaint D, Messika-Zeitoun D, Maalouf J, et al. Quantitive echocardiographic determinants of clinical outcome in asymptomatic patients with aortic regurgitation. A prospective study. J Am Coll Cardiol CVI. 2008;1(1):1–11.
15. Hamirini YS, Dietl CA, Voyles W, Peralta M, Begay D & Raizad V. Acute aortic regurgitation. Circulation 2012;126(9):1121–6.

Mitral Valve Disease 9

Mitral Stenosis

1. **Appearance of the valve, annulus and chords**
   - Mitral annulus calcification is increasingly common in our aging population. It usually causes no more than moderate stenosis. It may be misdiagnosed as severe mitral stenosis because:
     - The extensive annular calcification may be mistaken for valve calcification.
     - It may be hard to image the relatively thin and mobile mitral leaflets.
   - Stenosis of the mitral valve leaflets is usually rheumatic (Table 9.1). In early chronic disease, there is:
     - Commissural fusion ('fish mouth' appearance on the parasternal short-axis view).
     - Thickening of the leaflet tips ('drumstick' appearance) but thin and mobile leaflets.
   - In established rheumatic disease, there is progressive scarring and calcification. Describe:
     - The commissures. Are both fused? Is there calcium at the commissures? If so, is it in the outer part or the whole of the fused edge?
     - Leaflet thickening. Is it just at the tips, or does it extend over the whole leaflet or only a part?
     - Leaflet mobility. Often, the posterior leaflet is immobile, but the anterior leaflet still bows fully. Is the anterior leaflet less mobile or completely immobile?
     - The degree of chordal thickening and shortening. Are individual chords still visible? Are chords partially matted together? Do the chords form a secondary orifice, causing deviation or splitting of the colour profile within the LV? Is it impossible to see where the papillary muscles end and the chords begin?

Table 9.1 **Causes of mitral stenosis**

Common	Rheumatic disease, mitral annulus calcification
Uncommon	Radiation, systemic lupus erythematosus, congenital

DOI: 10.1201/9781003242789-9

101

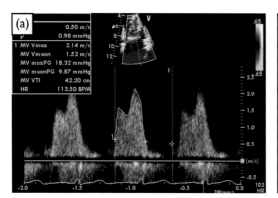

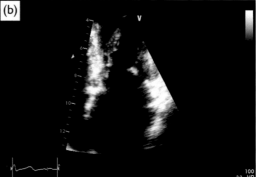

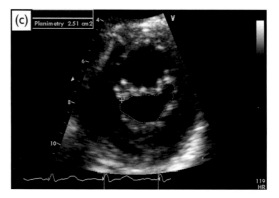

Figure 9.1 Pseudo-severe mitral stenosis. In patients with mitral annulus calcification, it is uncommon for the mitral stenosis to be severe. However, there may be a large A wave as a result of underlying LV diastolic dysfunction. This can increase the estimated transmitral gradient to levels suggesting severe stenosis despite a mild or moderate orifice area (b). In this example, the mean gradient is 9 mmHg (a) despite an orifice area 2.5 cm^2 (c).

And here's an electronic link to a loop on the website or use
http://goo.gl/EDsYfs

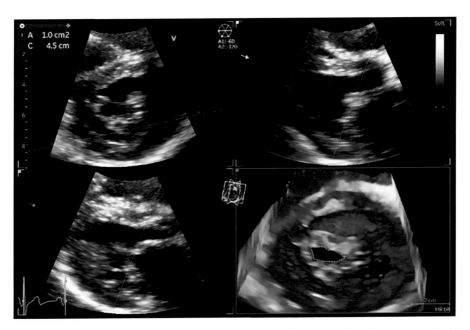

Figure 9.2 **Planimetry of the mitral orifice.** Care must be taken to section the tips of the mitral leaflets perpendicularly. This is aided by 3D. A common mistake is to section towards the base of the leaflets or across thickened chords.

2. Planimeter the orifice area

- Make sure that the section is not oblique. This is aided by 3D (Figure 9.2).
- Use colour Doppler as a guide to the extent of the orifice if this is not obvious on imaging.
- Take care not to include the chords, which, if thickened, can mimic the orifice.
- If there is significant thickening with reverberation artefact, the measurement may be inaccurate and should not be made.
- In mitral annulus calcification, planimetry is not valid or feasible. If colour flow through the valve is wide in all views with no major aliasing, then there is no significant stenosis.

3. Continuous wave signal

- Average the pressure half-time and mean gradient over three cycles. Choose cycles with an instantaneous heart rate close to 60–90 bpm if there is atrial fibrillation.
- There is little point in averaging many cycles if the heart rate is so high as to reduce mitral valve flow. Better to wait for rate control.
- The Hatle formula (orifice area = 220/pressure half-time) is an approximate guide to severity in moderate or severe stenosis.

- In mitral annulus calcification in sinus rhythm, a large transmitral A wave (Figure 9.1) causes overestimation using the grading thresholds derived from patients in atrial fibrillation. Some labs measure the gradient omitting the A wave, but individual cases may need MDT discussion using all TTE modalities, including qualitative assessment by colour Doppler.

4. **Assess mitral regurgitation** (see page 115)
   - Anything more than mild mitral regurgitation means that the valve is not suitable for balloon valvotomy.
   - The transmitral pressure half-time will be shortened disproportionate to the orifice area if there is severe mitral or aortic regurgitation.
   - The mean transmitral gradient will increase if there is significant mitral regurgitation (see Chapter 11).

5. **Grade the mitral stenosis** (Table 9.2)
   - The planimetered orifice area is the most reliable measure in rheumatic disease if performed accurately. The gradient and pulmonary artery pressure are flow-dependent.
   - Intervention is increasingly dominated by balloon valvotomy, which is usually more successful when the orifice area is <1.5 cm^2 and before the valve is severely calcified.

6. **Examine the right heart**
   - The pulmonary artery pressure (see Chapter 5) has a loose relationship with the severity of mitral stenosis. A pulmonary artery systolic pressure >50 mmHg at rest is a criterion for balloon valvotomy[2, 3].
   - RV dilatation with hypokinesis is a more important predictor of poor outcome at mitral valve surgery than the pulmonary artery pressure, which may fall after mitral valve replacement.

Table 9.2 **Criteria of severity in mitral stenosis[1]**

Measurement	Mild	Significant* Moderate	Significant* Severe
Orifice area by planimetry (cm^2)	>1.5	1.0–1.5	<1.0
Pressure half-time (ms)	<150	150–220	>220
Mean gradient (mmHg)	<5	5–10	>10+
PA pressure (mmHg)	<30	30–50	>50**

* 'Significant' is a term in the new guidelines[2, 3] meaning moderate or severe mitral stenosis.

+ >15 mmHg after exercise.

** The relationship with valve stenosis is not tight.

- Tricuspid rheumatic involvement is common but easily missed.
- More than mild tricuspid regurgitation with a tricuspid annulus diameter ≥40 mm (≥21 mm/m²) is currently an indication for tricuspid annuloplasty at the time of mitral valve replacement[4].

7. Assess the other valves

- Significant aortic valve disease may mean that double valve replacement rather than balloon mitral valvotomy is indicated.
- Aortic stenosis can be underestimated because of low flow caused by severe mitral stenosis (or regurgitation).

8. If the patient has symptoms but the orifice area is >1.5 cm²

Symptoms occur on exertion, but the TTE so far has been at rest.

- Ask the patient to exercise until breathless. This can be done on a bicycle or treadmill or, more simply, by walking around the echocardiography department then immediately getting back on the couch.
- A mean gradient >15 mmHg after exercise is an indication for considering balloon valvotomy[2, 3] (Table 9.3).

Table 9.3 **Guideline indications for intervention in mitral stenosis[2, 3]**

Symptoms	Orifice area	Extra	Intervention	Class
Y	≤1.5	Suitable for balloon	Balloon	I
Y	≤1.5	Not suitable	Surgery	I
N	≤1.5	PA pressure at rest >50 mmHg	Balloon	2a
N	≤1.5	Need for non-cardiac surgery or pregnancy	Balloon	2a
N	≤1.5	New AF (or dense contrast, prior embolism)	Balloon	2b
Y	>1.5	Exercise mΔP >15 mmHg or resting wedge >25 mmHg	Balloon	2b
Y	≤1.5	Not suitable for surgery and not ideal for balloon	Balloon	2b
N	≤1.5	LA volume >60 mL/m² and sinus rhythm	Warfarin	2a

Table 9.4 Markers of successful balloon valvotomy

Good mobility of the anterior leaflet
No more than minor chordal involvement (Figure 9.2)
No more than mild mitral regurgitation
No commissural calcification (Figure 9.2)
No left atrial thrombus (on TOE)

9. **Risk of atrial thrombus**
   - TTE is insensitive for detecting thrombus. A TOE should always be performed before balloon valvotomy.
   - A dilated left atrium (volume >60 mL/m^2) is a criterion for considering warfarin in moderate or severe mitral stenosis and sinus rhythm[2, 5].

10. **Is the valve suitable for balloon valvotomy?**
    - The most reliable characteristics of the valve for predicting success without developing severe mitral regurgitation are given in Table 9.4.
    - Some centres use the Wilkins system of scoring 1 to 4 for valve mobility, thickening, calcification, and subvalvular involvement[6] (Appendix Table A.6), with a score ≤8 suggesting that balloon valvotomy will be successful. This system does not focus on some important markers (Table 9.4), notably the site of commissural calcification.

⚠ MISTAKES TO AVOID

- Off-axis planimetry of the mitral valve.
- Failing to take account of the effects of severe MR or AR on transmitral pressure half-time.
- Overestimating the degree of stenosis in patients with a heavily calcified annulus in sinus rhythm because of a large A wave.

Mitral Regurgitation

1. **Appearance and movement of the valve**
   - MR is either primary (caused by an abnormality of the valve) or secondary (caused by LV dysfunction) (Table 9.5). In primary MR, the valve looks abnormal, while in secondary MR, the valve looks normal but is restricted ('tented') in systole (Table 9.5).

Table 9.5 **Causes of mitral regurgitation**

Cause	Valve appearance	Movement	Jet direction
Primary (organic) (i.e. abnormal mitral valve)			
Floppy mitral valve	Variable myxomatous change	Prolapse in systole	Away from prolapse
Rheumatic disease	Thickened tips	Bowing in diastole	Usually central
Endocarditis	Vegetation, destruction	Sections of valve may move out of phase	Variable
Other: SLE, drugs	Generalised thickening	Systolic restriction	Usually central
Secondary (functional) (i.e. abnormal LV)*			
Inferior or inferolateral infarct	Normal	Posterior restriction	Posterior
Inferior and anterior infarcts	Normal	Symmetrical restriction	Central
Global LV dilatation	Normal	Usually symmetrical restriction	Central

* Papillary muscle rupture is usually considered separately as acute ischaemic mitral regurgitation. 'Ischaemic mitral regurgitation' is used for secondary mitral regurgitation caused by myocardial infarction.

- The mitral valve apparatus consists of the leaflets, chords, annulus, and adjacent myocardium. However, the main clues to the aetiology are in the leaflets themselves (Table 9.5).

Appearance of the valve
- Thickened leaflet tips are typical of rheumatic disease, often with rigid posterior leaflet, commissural fusion, and chordal thickening and matting.
- Generalised thickening occurs in antiphospholipid syndrome or late after high-dose radiation or after drugs (e.g. cabergoline, pergolide, phentermine).
- A floppy valve may only look thickened as prolapse develops in systole and is often associated with lax chords and a dilated mitral annulus.
- A discrete mass attached to the leaflet suggests a vegetation.
- In the context of an acute coronary syndrome, consider a ruptured papillary muscle tip.
- A ruptured chord is usually a thin whip-like structure associated with prolapse.

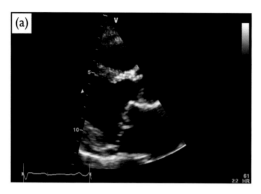 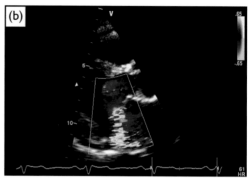

Figure 9.3 **Mitral prolapse.** In this image, the anterior leaflet prolapse (a) and the regurgitant jet is directed posteriorly (b), away from the abnormal leaflet.

Movement of the valve

- **Mitral prolapse is defined as:**
  - Movement of part of either leaflet >2 mm behind the plane of the annulus in the parasternal or apical long-axis views.
  - Displacement of the point of coaptation behind the plane of the annulus in the 4-chamber view.
- **However, prolapse of the medial or lateral parts of the leaflets may only be seen in other views:**
  - Prolapse of A3, P3, or the medial commissure may be seen in the apical 2-chamber view, the parasternal short-axis view, or the parasternal long-axis view tilted towards the RV.
  - Prolapse of A1, P1, or the lateral commissure may be seen in the apical 2-chamber view, the parasternal short-axis view, or the parasternal long-axis view tilted towards the pulmonary artery.
- **Is there evidence of prolapse?** (Figure 9.3)
  - anterior or posterior leaflets or both?
  - Which segments are involved using the Carpentier classification (Figure 9.4)?
  - Does prolapse affect the leaflet tip, the whole leaflet (like a bucket handle), or is it flail (moving through 180° and often with a visible ruptured chord)?
- **Is there restriction of opening in diastole?**
  - Restriction of both leaflet tips with doming of the rest of the leaflets occurs in rheumatic disease.
  - Confusion occasionally arises because of reduced opening of the whole of both leaflets (not just the tip) as a result of low cardiac output or of the anterior leaflet alone because of an impinging jet of aortic regurgitation.

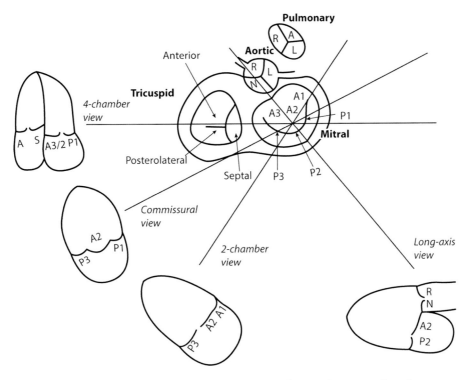

Figure 9.4 **Mitral valve segments on transthoracic examination.**

- **Is there restriction of both leaflets during systole (symmetrical tenting)?** (Figure 9.5)
  - This is usually associated with severe LV systolic dysfunction either a globally dilated and hypokinetic LV or myocardial infarction in both inferior and anterior territories.
  - The MR jet is directed centrally.

- **Is there restriction of the posterior leaflet during systole (asymmetrical tenting)?** (Figure 3.1)
  - This is usually associated with an inferior or inferolateral (posterior) infarction, sometimes affecting only a small section of myocardium, making it difficult to detect. Occasionally, it is caused by fibrotic shortening of the chords.
  - The restriction may be subtle.
  - The MR jet is directed posteriorly.

- **If the leaflets look and move normally:**
  - Check the annulus diameter. A diameter >35 mm in women and >40 mm in men raises the suspicion of dilatation[7]. Isolated annulus dilatation can cause severe MR even without leaflet prolapse or LV dysfunction.

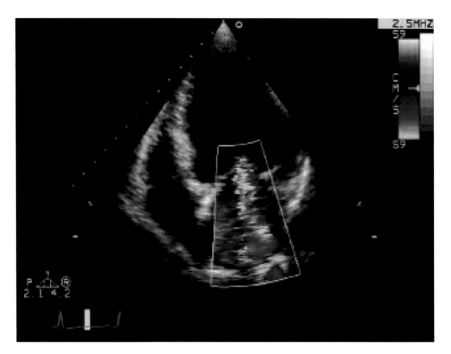

Figure 9.5 Secondary mitral regurgitation. In secondary regurgitation, as a result of symmetrical tenting of the leaflets, the regurgitant jet is central; if one leaflet is slightly more restricted than the other, the jet will be directed towards that leaflet.

Table 9.6 **Restricted leaflet motion**

Both leaflets
Tenting (point of apposition above the plane of the annulus in the 4-chamber view)
Centrally directed jet of regurgitation (Figure 9.5)
Dilated LV causing abnormal papillary muscle function
Restriction of posterior leaflet motion
Tip of leaflet held in LV during systole (best seen in a long-axis view) (Figure 3.1)
Jet directed posteriorly (Figure 3.1)
Inferior or inferolateral (posterior) infarct

- Check for a perforation or cleft.
- Check for commissural prolapse:
    - The jet origin will be to the medial or lateral part of the orifice in the parasternal short-axis view.
    - A jet from the commissure imaged in the parasternal long-axis view may be mistaken for a perforation.

- Angling from the parasternal long-axis view medially towards the RV will bring prolapse of the medial commissure into view. Angling laterally towards the PA will bring prolapse of the lateral commissure into view.

- The abnormality may be more obvious on 3D. If image quality is suboptimal, consider TOE.

2. Colour flow mapping

The following should be assessed[7]:

- The origin of the jet (e.g. medial, central, or lateral part of the orifice).
- The direction of the jet:
  - Away from a prolapsing leaflet (Figure 9.3b).
  - Behind a restricted leaflet (Figure 3.1b).
  - Centrally in symmetrical 'tenting' of the leaflets (Figure 9.5).

- The width of the jet at the level of the orifice using either:
  - The vena contracta width averaged from two orthogonal views, usually 4- and 3-chamber (or parasternal long-axis view) (Figure 9.6).
  - The PISA method (Figure 9.7).

- The size of the flow convergence zone within the left ventricle is assessed by eye.

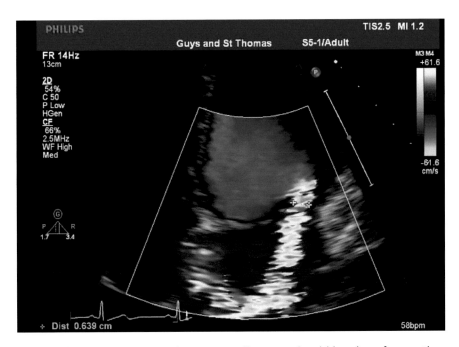

Figure 9.6 **Vena contracta.** An average diameter should be given from orthogonal views as many jets are oval in cross-section rather than circular.

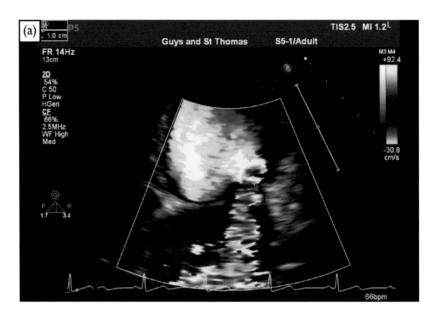

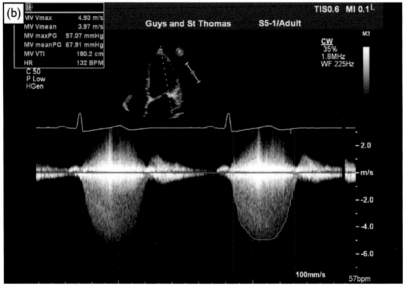

Figure 9.7 The PISA method.

1. Lower the image depth to increase the size of the area of interest.
2. Reduce the Nyquist limit to 15–40 cm/s.
3. Measure the radius of the first aliasing shell at mid-systole (V_a) (Figure 9.7a).
4. Measure the peak velocity (V_{cw}) and velocity time integral (VTI_{cw}) of the continuous wave mitral regurgitant signal (Figure 9.7b).
5. The formulae are:
   - EROA = 10 $(2\pi r^2 V_a/V_{cw})$
   - R Vol = (EROA $\times$ VTI_{cw})/100

- The duration of the jet using colour M-mode:
  - Is it holosystolic or present only in part of the systole, usually the latter part, as prolapse develops in bileaflet prolapse?
  - The quantification of a jet based on jet width or PISA has to be downgraded according to common-sense judgement if it is non-holosystolic.

3. **Continuous wave signal**
   - Look at the shape and density of the signal. A signal as dense as forward flow suggests severe regurgitation. A low-intensity or incomplete signal suggests mild regurgitation and an intermediate signal moderate regurgitation.
   - Rapid depressurisation causes a 'dagger-shaped' signal and is a sign of severe regurgitation.

4. **Pulsed Doppler**
   - Severe mitral regurgitation is suggested by:
     - A high transmitral E wave velocity (>1.5 m/s) in the absence of mitral stenosis.
     - A ratio of $VTI_{mitral}/VTI_{subaortic}$ >1.4.[7]
   - A pulsed sample in a pulmonary vein at a distance from the jet can aid quantification, although this is most useful on TOE. Blunting of the systolic signal occurs in moderate and severe regurgitation and flow reversal in very severe regurgitation.
   - The estimation of filling pressures using the E/E' ratio is not valid in the presence of severe mitral regurgitation.

5. **LV function**
   - Measure linear dimensions at the base of the heart. The systolic dimension is particularly important and should be averaged over several cycles.
   - In regurgitation caused by a floppy valve, surgery can be considered even in the absence of symptoms if the systolic dimension is ≥40 mm or the LV ejection fraction ≤60% and the valve is repairable at low risk.
   - LV shape may often change in severe MR, making linear dimensions unrepresentative of the whole LV. LV systolic volumes (biplane Simpson's method or 3D) then aid the detection of progressive LV dilatation on serial studies. There are no agreed cut points for surgery based on volumes.

6. **General**

Assess the left atrium
   - A dilated LA is a non-specific sign of chronic severe MR but also occurs in atrial fibrillation, systemic hypertension, or LV diastolic dysfunction.

- Progressive LA dilatation reaching an indexed volume >60 mL/m^2 is a secondary indication for surgery in an asymptomatic patient with a repairable mitral valve[2]. However, in practice it is almost never used alone.

Assess the right heart

- Pulmonary hypertension may complicate severe MR.
- A PA pressure >50 mmHg at rest is an indication for surgery in asymptomatic severe MR[2].

Assess the other valves

- The significance of aortic stenosis may be underestimated from the transaortic velocities as a result of low forward flow in severe mitral regurgitation.
- Tricuspid annuloplasty may be considered at the time of mitral valve surgery if there is mild or more tricuspid regurgitation and a tricuspid annulus diameter >40 mm.

7. **Grading regurgitation** (Table 9.7)

- Use all TTE modalities to grade the regurgitation.
- Multiple jets may be hard to quantify using jet characteristics alone. Use the indirect signs:
  - A hyperdynamic LV.
  - Pulmonary vein flow.
  - LA size (non-specific).
  - Pulmonary hypertension.

8. **Acute mitral regurgitation**

This is usually caused by papillary muscle rupture in acute myocardial infarction but can also occur after deceleration injury or chordal rupture in endocarditis.

It causes hypotension and pulmonary oedema, but there may be no murmur:

- The hyperdynamic LV is the major clue (but also occurs with post-infarct VSD).
- Because of the low LV pressure and high LA pressure, the jet momentum may fall quickly, resulting in a short colour flow signal, which may be missed. However, it will be broad and may fill the whole mitral annulus.
- There will be a to and fro signal throughout the cardiac cycle at the mitral annulus on a continuous wave or pulsed Doppler.
- A TOE (once the patient is ventilated) is often needed to confirm the diagnosis.

Table 9.7 **Grading mitral regurgitation**[7]

Measurement	Mild	Moderate	Severe
Neck width (mm)	<3	3–6.9	≥7
Flow convergence zone	Absent	Moderate	Large

PISA Quantities

Measurement	Mild	Mild-mod	Mod-severe	Severe
EROA (mm²)	<20	20–29	30–39	≥40
Regurgitant volume (mL)	<30	30–44	45–59	≥60
RF %	<30	30–39	40–49	≥50

Note: EROA effective regurgitant orifice area using PISA method.

 # MISTAKES TO AVOID

- A hyperdynamic LV suggests severe MR, so think twice before reporting mild or moderate MR.
- Missing early LV dysfunction because LV ejection fraction is in the low normal range for a LV with normal loading (Table 2.7).
- Missing papillary muscle rupture in haemodynamic deterioration after myocardial infarction.
- Mistaking posterior restriction for anterior prolapse (both cause a posteriorly directed jet of regurgitation).
- Excessive use of TOE when the information needed is obtainable on TTE.

CHECKLIST FOR REPORT IN MITRAL VALVE DISEASE

1. Detailed description of the valve appearance and movement, including mechanism of mitral disease (and, if possible, the cause).
2. Grade of stenosis and regurgitation.
3. LV dimensions, volume, and systolic function.
4. RV size and function, pulmonary artery pressure.
5. Tricuspid annulus diameter.
6. Left atrial size.
7. Presence of other valve disease.
8. For isolated mitral stenosis, is the valve suitable for balloon valvotomy?

Specialist Pre- and Post-Operative Assessment

1. Surgery in primary (organic) mitral regurgitation

- In asymptomatic patients with severe primary MR, the indications for surgery (Table 9.8) depend on LV systolic size and function and the likelihood of repair:

Table 9.8 **Indications for surgery in asymptomatic patients with severe primary mitral regurgitation**[2, 3]

Indications for surgery	Class
LVSD ≥40 mm or EF ≤ 60%	I
PA systolic pressure at rest >50 mmHg	2a
LA volume ≥60 mL/m²	2a
LVSD <40 mm and LVEF >60% if repair near certain at a 'valve centre of excellence'	2a

- **Likely**—localised prolapse, especially P2, or A2 (middle portion of posterior or anterior leaflets) or medial commissure or localised perforation.
- **Hard**—involvement of the whole of the posterior leaflet, destruction after endocarditis, rheumatic disease with pliable anterior leaflet, moderate or severe annular calcification, bileaflet prolapse.
- **Not likely**—extensive prolapse involving the anterior leaflet; rheumatic disease, especially with a rigid anterior leaflet; extensive destruction after endocarditis; extensive annular calcification.
- A tricuspid annuloplasty is usually performed at the time of mitral valve surgery if there is:
  - ≥ Moderate tricuspid regurgitation.
  - A combination of ≥ mild tricuspid regurgitation and a tricuspid annulus diameter ≥40 mm (≥21 mm/m²).
- Patients unfit for surgery may be considered for a transcatheter edge to edge repair procedure (TEER) in the absence of adverse features[7] (Table 9.9).

2. Surgery in secondary (functional) mitral regurgitation

- Management decisions are far harder than for primary mitral regurgitation because the underlying LV dysfunction may not improve after intervention and will also increase surgical risk.
- Intervention is only considered if the patient remains unwell after full medical therapy, including CRT, if appropriate.

Table 9.9 **Unfavourable features for TEER in primary and secondary MR**

Primary MR	Secondary MR
Leaflet perforation or large cleft	Severe tenting (coaptation depth >11 mm)
Rheumatic disease	Coaptation length <2 mm, large coaptation gap
Large flail gap >10 mm	Posterior leaflet length <7 mm
Large flail width >15 mm	LVDD >70 mm; LVEDV >200 mL or LVEDV index >96 mL/m^2
More moderate MR, EROA <30 mm^2*	
Mitral valve opening area ≤4.0 cm^2	
Leaflet calcification in the grasping area	

* The COAPT trial showed good results in patients with a mean indexed LV volume 101 mL/m^2 and MR EROA 41 mm^2, while the MITRA-FR trial had poor results in patients with a mean indexed LV volume 130 mL/m^2 and MR EROA 31 mm^2.

Table 9.10 **Adverse features for surgical repair[7] for secondary mitral regurgitation**

Left ventricle	Mitral valve
• LVDD >65 mm • LVSD >51 mm • LV systolic volume >140 mL • Interpapillary muscle distance >20 mm • Distance between base of posterior papillary muscle and fibrosa >40 mm • Sphericity index >0.7 • Lateral wall motion abnormality	• Broad, eccentric, or complex jet • Small or normal MV annulus, as a guide <35 mm • Tenting height >10 mm (area >1.6 cm^2) or posterior angle >45° • Heavy annular calcification

- A heart team must integrate the clinical features and echocardiogram. The decision is determined by LV function, the presence of myocardial viability (meaning, that LV function might improve after PCI or CABG), and the grade of MR and morphology of the mitral valve (Table 9.10) (Figure 9.8).

- Patients unsuitable for surgical repair may still benefit from valve replacement, and this is sometimes preferable to a repair since it needs a shorter operation and guarantees elimination of the MR.

- Stress echocardiography may be considered. Patients with leaflet tenting and ischaemic disease are more likely to increase the degree of mitral regurgitation on exercise[8].

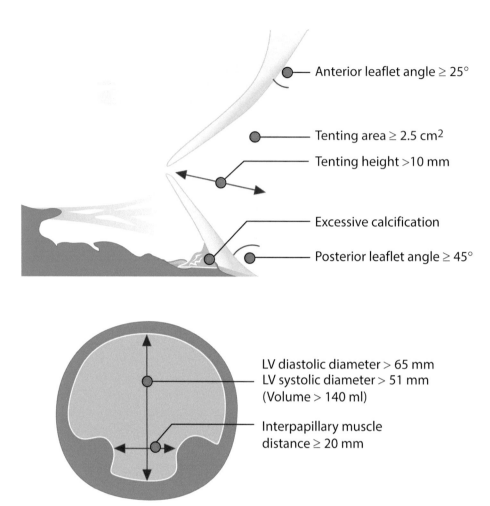

Anterior leaflet angle $\geq 25°$

Tenting area ≥ 2.5 cm^2
Tenting height >10 mm

Excessive calcification

Posterior leaflet angle $\geq 45°$

LV diastolic diameter > 65 mm
LV systolic diameter > 51 mm
(Volume > 140 ml)

Interpapillary muscle
distance ≥ 20 mm

Figure 9.8 Markers of a low likelihood of repair in secondary mitral regurgitation.

- Exercise echocardiography is indicated for:
  - Patients with breathlessness out of proportion to the grade of MR or LV dysfunction.
  - Patients with mild or moderate MR about to have CABG.
  - Acute pulmonary oedema with no known cause.
- Dobutamine stress echocardiography is indicated for patients with an impaired LV to determine whether there is evidence of viability.
- If a patient is judged too high risk for surgery, they may be considered for transcatheter edge-to-edge repair (TEER) in the absence of adverse characteristics (Table 9.9).

3. Echocardiography after mitral valve repair

A checklist after surgical repair and TEER is given in Table 9.11.

Table 9.11 **Echocardiography after mitral valve repair or TEER**

Appearance of the mitral valve, chords and annuloplasty ring or clips
Residual regurgitation • Grade • Localisation (middle, medial, lateral) • Through the valve or around the annuloplasty ring after surgical repair?
Presence and degree of mitral stenosis
Systolic anterior motion of the anterior leaflet? LV outflow acceleration
LV size and function
RV size and function and PA pressure
Left atrial size

3.1 Appearance

Surgical repairs may involve:

- Resection of valve tissue with reduction in the height of the leaflet. A shortened thickened immobile posterior echogenic structure is normal after P2 repair.
- Annuloplasty ring. Echogenic structure at the base of the leaflets.
- Artificial chords. These show as more dense than natural chords.
- Alfieri stitch. This is uncommon but is a stitch placed in the middle of the orifice, producing a double-orifice mitral valve.

After TEER, appearances include:

- Highly echogenic clips.
- For secondary MR, a single central clip may be placed, causing a double-orifice mitral valve.

Adverse features to assess:

- Stenosis of the native mitral valve.
- Systolic anterior motion of the anterior mitral leaflet causing LV outflow flow acceleration.
- Unsuccessful or partially successful procedure with residual MR.

References

1. Baumgartner H, Hung J, Bermejo J, et al. Echocardiographic assessment of valve stenosis: EAE/ASE Recommendations for clinical practice. Europ J Echo 2009;10:1–25.

2. Vahanian A, Beyersdorf F, Praz F, et al. 2021 ESC/EACTS Guidelines for the management of valvular heart disease. Eur Heart J 2022;43(7):561–632.
3. Otto CM, Nishimura RA, Bonow RO, et al. 2020 ACC/AHA Guideline for the management of patients with valvular heart disease: A report of the American College of Cardiology/American Heart Association Joint Committee on Clinical Practice Guidelines. Circulation 2021;143(5):e72–227.
4. Dreyfus GD, Corbi PJ, Chan KM & Bahrami T. Secondary tricuspid regurgitation or dilatation: Which should be the criteria for surgical repair? Ann Thorac Surg 2005;79(1):127–32.
5. Keenan NG, Cueff C, Cimidavella C, Brochet E, Lepage L, Detaint D, Himbert D, Iung B, Vahanian A & Messika-Zeitoun D. Usefulness of left atrial volume versus diameter to assess thromboembolic risk in mitral stenosis. Am J Cardiol 2010;106(8):1152–6.
6. Wilkins GT, Weyman AE, Abascal VM, Block PC & Palacios IF. Percutaneous balloon dilatation of the mitral valve: An analysis of echocardiographic variables related to outcome and the mechanism of dilatation. Brit Heart J 1988;60(4):299–308.
7. Lancellotti P, Pibarot P, Chambers J, et al. Multimodality imaging assessment of native valvular regurgitation: An EACVI and ESC Council of valvular heart disease position paper. Europ Heart J CVI 2022;23(5):e171–232.
8. Lancellotti P, Troisfontaines P, Toussaunt AC & Pierard LA. Prognostic importance of exercise-induced changes in mitral regurgitation in patients with chronic ischaemic left ventricular dysfunction. Circulation 2003;108(14):1713–7.

Right-Sided Valve Disease

10

The right-sided valves are assessed in the minimum standard TTE. Pay particular attention if there is:

- Left-sided disease.
- RV dilatation, especially if the RV is hyperdynamic.

Tricuspid Regurgitation

Trace or mild tricuspid regurgitation (TR) is normal and seen in 80% of studies. Steps to take if there is more than minor TR:

1. **Describe the appearance and movement of the valve**
   - Pathological TR is usually secondary (caused by dilatation of the RV or RA or by pulmonary hypertension), but it may be primary (caused by an abnormal valve) (Table 10.1).
   - Primary and secondary TR may coexist. Primary TR causing severe RV dilatation can lead to tethering of the valve and worsening TR.
   - Examine the valve in all views (Figure 10.1).
   - The normal apical displacement of the septal leaflet from the mitral annulus is up to 15 mm (indexed 8 mm/m^2).
   - The annulus is dilated if its diameter is ≥40 mm (21 mm/m^2) in the 4-chamber view[1].
   - Imaging all three leaflets is aided by 3D[2]. Preliminary 3D normal ranges for the annulus[3] are:
     - Long-axis 28–44 mm.
     - Short-axis 22–38 mm.
   - Progressive RV dilatation causes:
     - Initially, annular dilatation with failure of leaflet coaptation.
     - Further RV dilatation causes restriction of the leaflet tips.

2. **Grading TR**
   - Use all modalities available (Table 10.2). The most useful are the colour width and density of the continuous wave signal. Systolic flow reversal in the hepatic vein and IVC is specific for severe TR.

DOI: 10.1201/9781003242789-10

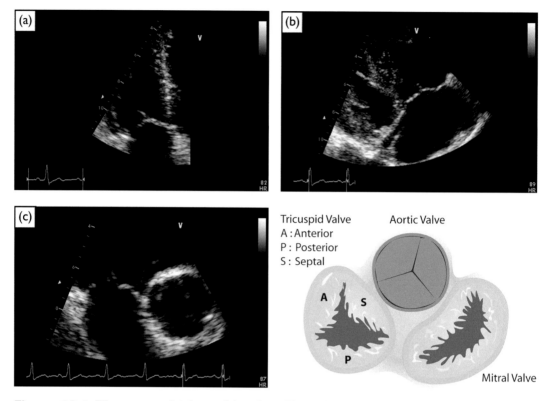

Figure 10.1 The normal tricuspid valve. The 4-chamber view (a) shows the anterior (left) and septal (right) leaflets. The parasternal long-axis view (b) shows the anterior (right) and either septal or posterior leaflet (left), depending on whether the septum or posterior LV wall is imaged. The short-axis view (c) shows the septal or anterior leaflet (right) and the anterior or posterior leaflet (left), depending on the cut.

Table 10.1 **Causes of tricuspid valve disease**

Cause	Notes
Primary	
Rheumatic disease	Doming without significant thickening. Commissural fusion may be more obvious on 3D. Associated left-sided rheumatic disease.
Floppy valve	Eccentric jet directed away from the prolapsing leaflet. Often associated with mitral prolapse.
Annular dilatation	May occur without prolapse. Associated with RA dilatation. The normal annulus diameter is <40 mm (<21 mm/m^2).
Endocarditis	May complicate IV drug use or indwelling venous cannulae.

Table 10.1 (Continued)

Cause	Notes
Carcinoid	Associated with pulmonary valve involvement. Fibrotic, stubby rigid leaflets.
Congenital	Ebstein's anomaly (see Table 16.8).
Drugs (e.g. pergolide)	General thickening and tenting.
Pacemaker	The electrode causes perforation, interferes with closure, adheres to the leaflet, or causes leaflet thickening.
Trauma	Prolapse with ruptured chords after blunt chest injury.
Iatrogenic	Endocardial biopsy can damage the valve or chords.
Secondary	
RV myopathy/RV infarct	Initially causes annular dilatation with failure of leaflet coaptation. If severe, causes leaflet restriction. Look for associated left-sided myocardial abnormalities.
Pulmonary hypertension	May be no abnormality of the leaflets, unless there is secondary RV dilatation.
Left-to-right shunts	An ASD causes RV volume overload.
RA dilatation	Chronic AF can cause tricuspid annulus dilatation as part of general RA dilatation.

Table 10.2 **Grading tricuspid regurgitation[4]**

	Mild	Moderate	Severe**
Colour neck (mm)	Usually none, but always <3	<7	≥7**
PISA radius (mm)	<6	6–9	>9
EROA (mm²)	–	–	≥40*
R vol (mL)	–	–	≥40*
Continuous wave	Incomplete	Low or mod intensity	Dense and may be triangular (Figure 10.2)
Hepatic vein flow	Normal	Maybe systolic blunting	Systolic reversal

* Not routinely performed.

** New grades are now established[4, 5]: severe 7–13 mm, massive 14–20 mm, and torrential ≥21 mm. These make clinical sense and help demonstrate the benefit of transcatheter techniques, which improve the grade of TR from torrential down to severe. This change would not register on the traditional grading scheme.

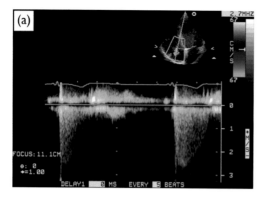
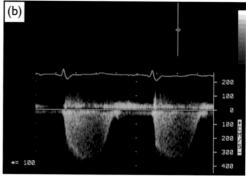
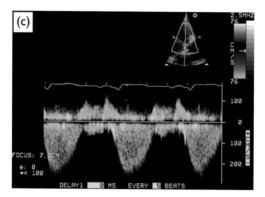

Figure 10.2 **Tricuspid regurgitation.** Mild regurgitation causes a dagger-shaped, low-intensity signal (a). Moderate regurgitation causes a large intratrial jet on colour mapping with a complete continuous wave signal (b). Severe regurgitation has a dense signal which initially retains its usual shape but, when very severe, may be dagger-shaped (c).

- Trivial or mild TR could be noted in the text but should not appear in the conclusion of the report. This might suggest significant valve disease to a non-echocardiographer.

3. **Describe RV size and function** (Chapter 4)
   - Progressive RV dilatation or reduction in systolic function are indications for surgery even without symptoms[2] in severe primary TR.
   - Early repair is recommended with a flail tricuspid leaflet after trauma if the RV is significantly dilated at the initial assessment but no thresholds are available[6].

4. **Estimate pulmonary artery pressure** (Chapter 5)

5. **Echocardiography and surgery**
   - Indications for surgery are in Table 10.3.
   - The type of surgery is guided by echocardiography.
   - Annular dilatation usually responds to annuloplasty.

Table 10.3 **Echocardiographic indications for surgery in severe tricuspid regurgitation[2]**

Primary tricuspid regurgitation
Severe TR and symptoms
Consider if severe TR and progressive dilatation and reduced function of the RV even with no symptoms
Having left-sided surgery
Moderate or worse TR
Mild TR and tricuspid annulus diam $\geq$40 mm ($\geq$21 mm/m^2)

- Severe systolic restriction usually requires more advanced repair techniques or valve replacement.
- Tricuspid prolapse may be repairable.
- Severe thickening usually suggests replacement rather than repair will be needed.

Tricuspid Stenosis

1. **Appearance of the valve**
   - TS is usually rheumatic but may also be congenital (Ebstein, tricuspid atresia) or occur in carcinoid or as a result of dense fibrosis secondary to SLE or multiple pacemaker electrodes.

2. **Recognising tricuspid stenosis**
   - Restriction of the leaflets (Figure 10.3) may not be obvious on imaging. Tricuspid stenosis is suggested if:
     - V_{max} >1.0 m/s (or more specific >1.5 m/s)[8]
     - Mean gradient >2 mmHg[9,10]
   - Signs suggesting severe stenosis are[2]:
     - Mean gradient $\geq$5 mmHg
     - Pressure half-time $\geq$190 ms
   - Another clue to severe tricuspid stenosis is a small RV (because of underfilling) and large RA (because of high back pressure).

3. **Surgery**
   - Surgery is indicated for severe tricuspid stenosis and symptoms or is performed at the time of surgery for coexistent left-sided disease.

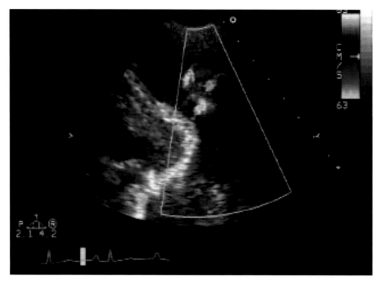

Figure 10.3 Tricuspid stenosis. Tricuspid stenosis may be missed because, unlike the situation with the mitral valve, there may be little thickening or calcification.

 ## MISTAKES TO AVOID

- A rheumatic tricuspid valve is easily missed because the leaflets can be thin. It rarely occurs alone, so always check the tricuspid valve if there is left-sided rheumatic disease.

CHECKLIST FOR THE REPORT IN TRICUSPID VALVE DISEASE

1. Tricuspid valve appearance and movement. Annulus diameter.
2. Grade of regurgitation.
3. Trans-tricuspid gradient if valve-restricted.
4. RV size and function and PA pressure.
5. Left-sided valves.

Pulmonary Stenosis and Regurgitation

- Pulmonary stenosis is almost always congenital (Table 10.4)[11]. It may be part of more complex cardiac lesions, especially tetralogy of Fallot, or associated with other lesions, for example, ASD. It may also be associated with more general congenital syndromes (Noonan, Williams, LEOPARD; see Table 16.1, page 172).

Table 10.4 **Causes of pulmonary valve disease**

Pulmonary stenosis	Pulmonary regurgitation
Congenital	Prior intervention for congenital stenosis
Carcinoid	Endocarditis
	Secondary • Pulmonary hypertension • PA or annular dilatation
	Carcinoid

● The obstruction is at valve level in 90%, subvalvar in 5%, supravalvar in 1%, and in a branch in 5%.

1. Appearance of the valve
  ● An initial clue to the presence of stenosis is turbulent flow in the RV outflow tract during systole on colour Doppler.
  ● A stenotic valve is either:
    ● Dysplastic and thickened (e.g. in Noonan syndrome)
    ● Relatively thin, but with systolic bowing, and therefore visible in systole as well as diastole

2. Is there pulmonary regurgitation?
  ● Trace or mild regurgitation is normal. A jet originating near the edge of the orifice should not be mistaken for coronary artery flow.
  ● Severe regurgitation is suggested by the findings in Table 10.5.

3. What is the pressure difference across the valve?
The main method of grading is by the transpulmonary V_{max} (Table 10.6)[11, 12].

Table 10.5 **Factors suggesting severe pulmonary regurgitation[4]**

A wide colour jet (e.g. >7.5 mm or >65% of the annulus diam)
Diastolic flow reversal visible in the distal main pulmonary artery or branches (Figure 10.4)
A steep dense continuous wave signal (pressure half-time <100 ms and deceleration time <260 ms) (Figure 10.5)
Ratio of PR duration:diastolic duration <0.77
Dilated, active RV

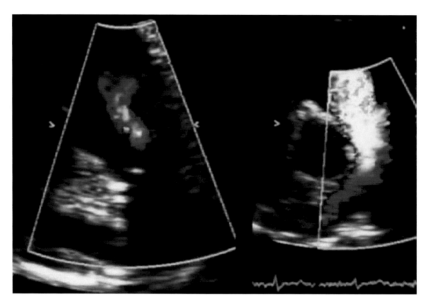

Figure 10.4 Pulmonary regurgitation—colour map. Mild regurgitation is shown on the left with a narrow jet originating at the valve level. Severe regurgitation on the right has a jet filling the RV outflow tract with flow reversal as far as the right pulmonary artery branch.

 And here's an electronic link to a loop on the website or use
http://goo.gl/eQmasZ

4. **Check the level of the obstruction**
   - A muscular obstruction in the RV outflow tract (infundibulum) or mid-cavity (double-chamber RV) may be mistaken for or be associated with pulmonary valve stenosis.
     - The continuous Doppler waveform may have a late-systolic peak but may also be identical to obstruction at valve level.
     - Pulsed Doppler may identify the level of obstruction.
     - The diagnosis commonly needs CMR if TTE image quality is suboptimal.
   - A pulmonary artery membrane may be mistaken for valve obstruction but is rare.

5. **What is pulmonary artery pressure?** (See Chapter 5)
   - Dominant PR may be caused by pulmonary hypertension.
   - PS protects the pulmonary circulation against the effect of high flow from a left-to-right shunt.

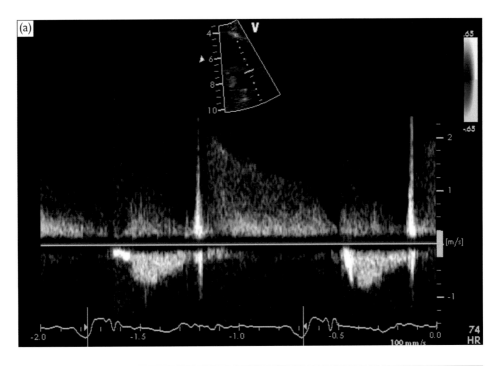

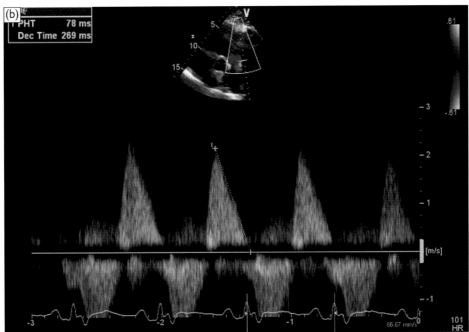

Figure 10.5 **Pulmonary regurgitation—continuous wave signal.** In normal mild PR, the signal has a slow descent (a), while in severe regurgitation (b), the pressure half-time is <100 ms, 78 ms in this example.

Table 10.6 **Grading pulmonary stenosis**

	Mild	Moderate	Severe
V_{max}	<3.0 m/s	3.0–4.0 m/s	>4.0 m/s
Peak gradient	<36 mmHg	36–64 mmHg	>64 mmHg

Table 10.7 **Guide to upper limit of normal pulmonary artery dimensions[13]**

RV outflow diameter (mm)	34
PV annulus (mm)	22
Main pulmonary artery (mm)	29
Right pulmonary branch (mm)	17
Left pulmonary branch (mm)	14

6. **Assess the pulmonary artery**
   - Look for dilatation of the main and branch pulmonary arteries. Little modern data exist, and Table 10.7 gives information on upper limits from 1984 as a guide.

7. **Assess RV size and function** (See Chapter 4)

8. **Other imaging modalities**
Once severe pulmonary valve disease is detected by echocardiography, **CMR** is used to:
   - Quantify the degree of PR. A regurgitant volume of >40 mL/beat and a regurgitant fraction >35% are thresholds for severe.
   - Measure RV volumes for serial studies.
   - Differentiate double-chamber RV (mid-cavity) from infundibular (RVOT) stenosis.
   - Assess branch pulmonary artery stenoses and lung perfusion.

9. **Are there indications for invasive intervention?**
   - If balloon valvotomy is feasible this can be considered if V_{max} >4.0 m/s even in the absence of symptoms[11].
   - If surgical valve replacement is needed, intervention should be discussed at an MDT if there is severe (or moderate) PS[11] or severe PR and:
     - Symptoms or reduced exercise tolerance.
     - A serial decrease in RV systolic function and progression of TR to ≥ moderate.
     - RV systolic pressure >80 mmHg (in PS).
     - Right-to-left shunting via an ASD or VSD (in PS).

MISTAKES TO AVOID

- Do not use the TR V_{max} alone to calculate PA systolic pressure if there is PS or other RV outflow obstruction. Subtracting the $4V^2_{pulm}$ from $4V^2_{tr}$ will give a better estimate.
- Missing severe PR because the diastolic jet may be wide and low momentum.

CHECKLIST FOR THE TTE IN PULMONARY VALVE DISEASE

1. Appearance and motion of the pulmonary valve.
2. V_{max} and mean gradient.
3. Grade of PR.
4. RV size, morphology and systolic function.
5. Diameter of pulmonary artery and estimated PA systolic pressure, if possible.

References

1. Vahanian A, Beyersdorf F, Praz F, et al. 2021 ESC/EACTS Guidelines for the management of valvular heart disease. Eur Heart J 2022;43(7):561–632.
2. Badano LP, Agricola E, de Isla LP, Gianfagna P & Zamorano JL. Evaluation of the tricuspid valve morphology and function by transthoracic real-time three-dimensional echocardiography. Europ J Echo 2009;10(4):477–84.
3. Addetia K, Muranu D, Veronesi F, et al. 3-Dimensional echocardiographic analysis of the tricuspid annulus provides new insights into right ventricular geometry and dynamics. J Am Coll Cardiol CVI 2019;12(3):401–12.
4. Lancellotti P, Pibarot P, Chambers J, et al. Multimodality imaging assessment of native valvular regurgitation: An EACVI and ESC Council of valvular heart disease position paper. Europ Heart J CVI 2022;23(5):e171–232.
5. Hahn RT, Zamorano JL. The need for a new tricuspid regurgitation grading scheme. Europ Heart J CVI 2017;18(12):1342–43.
6. Messika-Zeitoun. Medical and surgical outcome of tricuspid regurgitation caused by flail leaflets. J Thorac Cardiovasc Surg 2004;128(2):296–302.
7. Otto CM, Nishimura RA, Bonow RO, et al. 2020 ACC/AHA Guideline for the management of patients with valvular heart disease: A report of the American

College of Cardiology/American Heart Association Joint Committee on Clinical Practice Guidelines. Circulation 2021;143(5):e72–227.

8. Parris TM, Panidis JP, Ross J & Mintz GS. Doppler echocardiographic findings in rheumatic tricuspid stenosis. Am J Cardiol 1987;60(16):1414–6.

9. Ribeiro PA, Al Zaibag M, Al Kasab S, Hinchcliffe M, Halim M, Idris M, et al. Provocation and amplification of the transvalvular pressure gradient in rheumatic tricuspid stenosis. Am J Cardiol 1988;61(15):1307–11.

10. Fawzy ME, Mercer EN, Dunn B, Al-Amri M & Andaya W. Doppler echocardiography in the evaluation of tricuspid stenosis. Europ Heart J 1989;10(11):985–90.

11. Baumgartner H, de Backer J, Babu-Narayan SV, et al. 2020 ESC Guideline for the management of adult congenital heart disease. Europ Heart J 2021;42(6):563–645.

12. Stout KK, Daniel CJ, Abdoulhosu JA, et al. 2018 AHA/ACC Guidelines for the management of adults with congenital heart disease. Circulation 2019;139(14):e698–800.

13. Triulzi MO, Gillam LD & Gentile F. Normal adult cross-sectional echocardiographic values: Linear dimensions and chamber areas. Echocardiography 1984;1(4):403–26.

Mixed Valve Disease

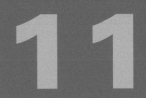

- This is increasingly common and was seen in 25% of patients in the 2017 European Heart Valve Survey[1].
- If one valve lesion is severe and the other only mild or moderate, then the severe lesion dominates management (see Chapters 8 and 9).
- Tricuspid regurgitation combined with left-sided disease is discussed in Chapter 10.
- For moderate mixed valve lesions, the key to assessment and management is:
  - The effect on the LV
  - The presence of symptoms
- If you are uncertain, bring the case to an MDT discussion.

Mixed Moderate Aortic Valve Disease

- The transaortic V_{max} gives a better assessment of overall severity than EOA.
- A V_{max} >4.0 m/s implies severe mixed disease even if the EOA is >1.0 cm^2.
- Surgery is indicated for symptoms.
- In the absence of symptoms, surgery should be considered if the LV ejection fraction is <50% or has reduced progressively on serial studies. No formal guideline thresholds exist[2].

Mixed Moderate Mitral Valve Disease

- Mixed disease occurs in rheumatic disease and increasingly as a result of mitral annulus calcification.
- A high transmitral gradient, whether caused by severe pure MS or mixed moderate disease, is still haemodynamically important. Management should be judged on symptoms and the haemodynamic effects on the RV and PA pressure.
- More than mild MR is a contraindication to balloon mitral valvotomy.

DOI: 10.1201/9781003242789-11

Mixed Mitral and Aortic Valve Disease

- Causes of confusion to guard against are:
  - Severe AR causes shortening of the transmitral pressure half-time in MS.
  - The jet of severe AR impinging on the anterior mitral leaflet can cause functional MS in the presence of an otherwise-normal mitral valve.
  - An eccentric jet of MR directed parallel to the LVOT can cause a CW signal similar to severe AS.
  - Reduced flow to the LVOT as a result of severe MS or MR is a cause of low-flow, low-gradient AS leading to potential underestimation of the severity of AS (see page 86).
  - Moderate AR and moderate MR together can cause severe LV volume load. Management is guided by symptoms and LV geometry and function and should be discussed at an MDT.
  - The assessment of MR in patients with severe AS is described on page 88. In general, mitral valve intervention is indicated by:
    - Primary disease of the mitral valve, for example, prolapse.
    - Moderate to severe or severe secondary MR.

References

1. Iung B, Delgado V, Rosenhek R, et al. Contemporary presentation and management of valvular heart disease. The Eurobservational Research Programme Valvular Heart Disease II Survey. Circulation 2019;140(14):1156–69.
2. Vahanian A, Beyersdorf F, Praz F, et al. 2021 ESC/EACTS Guidelines for the management of valvular heart disease. Eur Heart J 2022;43(7):561–632.

Prosthetic Heart Valves

12

- The core information to be gathered[1–3] is:
  - Appearance of the valve
  - Colour Doppler forward flow and regurgitation
  - Spectral Doppler
- The types of valve and their TTE features are given in Table 12.1 (see also Figure 12.1).

Core Information

1. **Appearance of the valve**
   - On imaging, prosthetic valves can be classed as normal (thin and mobile biological cusps) or failing (thick and restricted cusps or mechanical occluder):
     - The cusps of an AVR or TAVI are often best imaged from the apical long-axis view and a tricuspid prosthetic valve from a modified parasternal long-axis view.
     - The cage of an aortic caged-ball valve is also best seen in the apical long-axis view. A tilting disc or ball may both appear as an indistinct mass in a parasternal long-axis view and may be difficult to tell apart.
   - If image quality is suboptimal, colour Doppler filling the whole orifice in all views suggests normal opening.
   - Some appearances in a mitral valve which are normal but can cause confusion are:
     - The leaflets of a bileaflet mechanical valve may shut at slightly different rates.
     - Cavitations (bubbles) in the LV which occur with all types of valve but especially bileaflet mechanical valves.
     - Fibrin strands attached to the valve (seen best on TOE) are far thinner than vegetations and have no pathological significance.
     - If the surgeon has retained the posterior leaflet, a normal prosthetic mitral valve may rock slightly. In other positions, rocking suggests a large paraprosthetic leak. The diagnosis is established with colour Doppler.

DOI: 10.1201/9781003242789-12

Table 12.1 **Types of prosthetic valves**

Types	Makes	Common TTE features
SURGICALLY IMPLANTABLE BIOLOGICAL		
Stented animal tissue ('xenograft')		
Porcine	Duraflex, Mosaic, Epic, Hancock, Abbot (previously St Jude Medical), Biocor/ Labcor Porcine	Three 'crowns' of the stent and echogenic sewing ring, three thin and mobile cusps, trivial regurgitation through is normal.
Pericardial	Edwards Perimount/ Magna/Inspiris, Mitroflow, Labcor Pericardial, Biocor Pericardial, Trifecta, C-E Biophysio, Sorin More, Sorin Soprano	Ditto.
Sutureless	Perceval S, Edwards Intuity, 3F Enable, Trilogy	Ditto.
Stentless		
Porcine	Toronto, Medtronic Freestyle, Cryolife-O'Brien,* Koehler Elan, Labcor Stentless, Edwards Prima, Biocor	Some designs have prominent sewing cuffs, three thin and mobile cusps, trivial regurgitation through is normal.
Pericardial	Freedom Solo, Pericarbon	Three thin and mobile cusps, trivial regurgitation.
Homograft		May look like a normal native valve.
Ross procedure		Autograft may look like a normal native valve. Homograft in pulmonary position.
SURGICALLY IMPLANTED MECHANICAL		
Caged ball	Starr-Edwards	Cage may be hard to image in aortic position best seen in apical long-axis. Obvious in mitral position. Prominent reverberations from ball into LA. Mild central regurgitation is normal.

Stentless (Continued)		
Tilting disc	Bjork-Shiley,* Medtronic Hall, Sorin Allcarbon, Omnicarbon, Koehler Ultracor	Single disc obvious in MVR, may be mistaken for a mass in AVR. Regurgitation from major and minor orifices (through the disc for Medtronic-Hall).
Bileaflet	Abbot (previously St Jude), Carbomedics, On-X, Sorin Bicarbon, ATS, Medtronic Advantage, Edwards Mira	Visualisation of both leaflets easy in MVR and AVR depending on surgical orientation. Minor regurgitation at both pivots and occasionally around leaflets. Large 'bubbles' normal in the LV with MVR. Fibrin strands normal.
TRANSCATHETER		
Balloon-expandable	Edwards SAPIEN, SAPIEN XT, SAPIEN3	Short echogenic stent. Cusps difficult to image except in apical views. Mild regurgitation through is common.
Self-expandable	Medtronic CoreValve and Engager, Boston Scientific Lotus, Abbot Portico, Symetis Acurate, Direct Flow, Jena	Long echogenic stent. Cusps best imaged in apical views. Mild regurgitation through and around the valve is common.

Abbreviation: C-E Carpentier-Edwards.

* Now withdrawn.

2. **Colour Doppler**
   - All mechanical valves have 'physiological' regurgitation through the valve (Figure 12.2). These are narrow, with little or no aliasing. Regurgitation across the valve also occurs in about 10% of normal biological valves and is common in transcatheter valves.
   - **Paraprosthetic regurgitation is abnormal:**
     - Mild paraprosthetic regurgitation (best seen on TOE) can cause haemolysis. If asymptomatic, should be followed at least once after the baseline TTE to exclude progression.
     - In the mitral and tricuspid positions, an easily seen jet is usually paraprosthetic since normal transprosthetic regurgitation tends to be hidden by flow shielding (unless the LA is very large).
     - The intraventricular flow recruitment region of paraprosthetic regurgitation can usually be seen even when the intra-atrial jet is

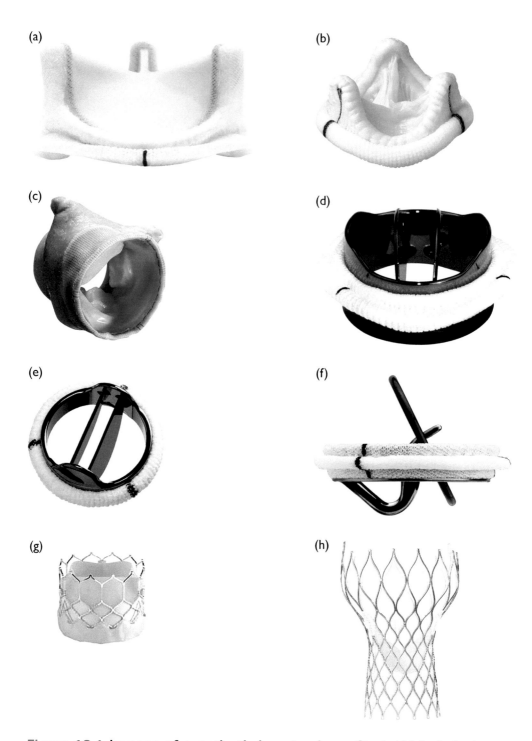

Figure 12.1 **Images of prosthetic heart valves.** *Stented biological valves*:
(a) Magna-Ease (bovine pericardial), (b) Epic (porcine). *Stentless biological valve*:
(c) Medtronic Freestyle. *Bileaflet mechanical mitral valve*: (d) OnX, (e) Abbot Master HP.
Single tilting disc: (f) Medtronic-Hall. *Transcatheter*: (g) Edwards SAPIEN, (h) Medtronic
Corevalve.

Long Axis **Short Axis**

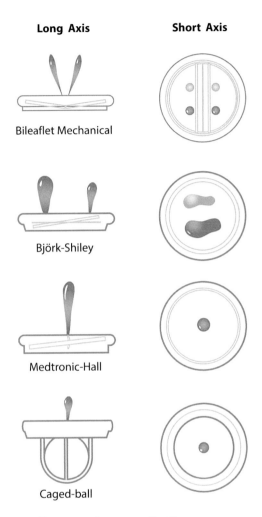

Bileaflet Mechanical

Björk-Shiley

Medtronic-Hall

Caged-ball

Figure 12.2 **Patterns of normal regurgitation.**

invisible. This allows the regurgitation to be localised using the sewing ring as a clockface.

- If there is doubt about the origin or size of a jet, TOE is indicated.

3. **Spectral Doppler**

- Steerable CW from the apex is sufficient if the patient is well and the valve clearly normal, but if there is doubt, the stand-alone probe should be used in at least two windows for an AVR.
- It is important not to position the pulsed sample too close to the AVR or TAVI, which results in an artefactually high EOA.
- The minimum dataset[1] is:
  - Aortic: V_{max}, mean gradient, and EOA using the continuity equation.

- Pulmonary: V_{max} and mean gradient.
- Mitral and tricuspid: Mean gradient, pressure half-time.

- For prosthetic mitral valves:
  - The Hatle formula (220/pressure half-time) is not valid.
  - The EOA and DVI are not routinely calculated but are used if uncertainty remains after imaging and basic spectral Doppler:
    - Mitral EOA is $CSA_{Ao} \times VTI_{subaortic}/VTI_{mitral.}$
    - Mitral DVI is $VTI_{mitral}/VTI_{subaortic}$ (ratio rises with obstruction).

- For aortic prosthetic valves, the aortic DVI may be useful as an adjunct if the LVOT diameter is hard to measure:
  - Aortic DVI is $VTI_{subaortic}/VTI_{Ao}$ (ratio falls with obstruction).

Is There Dysfunction of the Prosthetic Valve?

Patients may present with symptoms as a result of:

- Dysfunction of the prosthetic valve, causing regurgitation or obstruction (Table 12.2).
- Other structural cardiac disease: LV or RV dysfunction or other valve disease.

Table 12.2 Complications of prosthetic heart valves

Complication	Mechanical	Biological	Echocardiographic effect
Structural valve degeneration (SVD)	–	++++	Thickened cusps with regurgitation >> obstruction
Thrombosis	++	+	Obstruction
Thromboembolism	+++	+++	Nil
Infective endocarditis	++	++	Vegetations, abscess, new dehiscence
Pannus	+	+	Obstruction of closure or opening of leaflet; may be intermittent.
Dehiscence	++	++	Paraprosthetic regurgitation
Bleeding	+++	++	Nil

Note: + rare, ++ uncommon, +++ common, ++++ universal in long-lived patients, and – almost never occurs.

Echocardiography is important in differentiating these causes.
The key questions as you scan are:

1.   **Is the valve normal, or are there signs of early failure?**
2.   **If the V_{max} is high, is it from patient–prosthesis mismatch or obstruction?**
3.   **Is there regurgitation, and is it pathological?**
4.   **Is there other disease?**

1.   **Is the valve normal, or are there signs of early failure?**
   - Failure (structural valve deterioration or SVD) is inevitable in all biological valves and TAVI, if the patient lives sufficiently long, but almost never occurs in mechanical valves.
   - Early failure starts with thickening of the cusps and usually progresses gradually to cause obstruction or regurgitation. Occasionally, a tear in the base of the cusp can extend suddenly.
   - In practice, mild thickening and regurgitation is a prompt to consider annual echocardiograms. Moderate SVD (Tables 12.3 and 12.4) might prompt more frequent reassessment, depending on the clinical situation.
   - Re-intervention is indicated mainly for symptoms. In routine clinical practice, changes in valve morphology and haemodynamic function from baseline should be highlighted. Severe valve failure should be highlighted to the clinician in charge of the case (Tables 12.3 for surgical and transcatheter aortic valves and 12.4 for mitral valves).

2.   **High V_{max}. Patient–prosthesis mismatch vs obstruction**
   - All prosthetic valves are obstructive compared with a normal native valve because of the presence of a stent and sewing ring and the reduced compliance of the leaflet tissue.
   - Mild patient prosthesis mismatch is therefore normal, but severe mismatch may affect outcomes and cause symptoms[5].

Table 12.3 Guideline grading structural valve deterioration[4] in aortic surgical and transcatheter valves compared to a baseline study 1–3 months after surgery

	Mild	Moderate	Severe
Morphology	Thickening of the leaflets		
Obstruction	No significant change	↑ mean gradient ≥10 mmHg to ≥20 mmHg and ↓ EOA ≥0.3 cm² or ≥25% (or ↓ DVI ≥0.1 or ≥20%)	↑ mean gradient ≥20 mmHg to ≥30 mmHg and ↓ EOA ≥0.6 cm² or ≥50% (or ↓ DVI ≥0.2 or ≥40%)
Regurgitation through the valve	No significant change	↑ by ≥1 grade to ≥ moderate	↑ by ≥2 grades to severe

Table 12.4 Guideline grading structural valve deterioration[4] in biological mitral valves compared to a baseline study 1–3 months after surgery

	Mild	Moderate	Severe
Morphology	Thickening of the leaflets		
Obstruction	No significant change	↑ mean gradient ≥5 mmHg and ↑ DVI ≥0.4 or ≥20%, resulting in a DVI ≥2.2 (EOA ≥ 0.5 cm² or ≥25%)	↑ mean gradient ≥10 mmHg and ↑ DVI ≥0.8 or ≥40%, resulting in a DVI ≥2.7 (or EOA ≥1.0 cm² or ≥ 50% resulting in EOA <1.0 cm²)
Regurgitation through the valve	No significant change	↑ by ≥1 grade to ≥ moderate	↑ by ≥2 grades to ≥ moderate-severe

- The key features of patient–prosthesis mismatch are (Table 12.5 and Figure 12.3):
  - Normal valve appearance.
  - V_{max}, gradient, and EOA in normal range for valve design and size (Appendix Tables A.8-A.10).
  - No significant change in spectral Doppler from baseline study.
  - Low EOA indexed to BSA (Table 12.5).
- If the cusps or leaflets are not imaged well on TTE, consider:
  - TOE, but the leaflets of a mechanical valve may still be difficult to image.
  - Fluoroscopy.
  - CT, which may also image pannus.

Table 12.5 Differentiating patient–prosthesis mismatch from obstruction in aortic prosthetic valves

Key features	Patient–prosthesis mismatch	Obstruction
Appearance of the valve	Thin mobile cusps Colour fills orifice in all views	Cusps or disc thickened or reduced opening Restricted colour across the valve
Normal range spectral Doppler	Within for size and type of valve	Outside
Change from baseline - *Mean gradient* - *EOA*	≤10 mmHg* No change	>10 mmHg ↓ >0.3 cm²

* Mean gradient may rise if LV systolic dysfunction recovers after surgery, but the EOA should stay approximately constant.

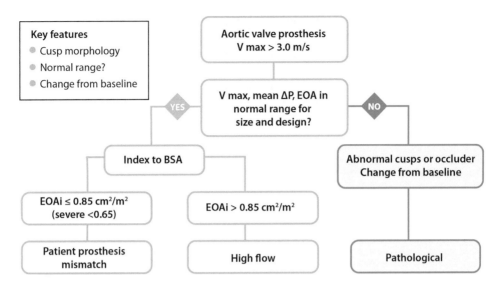

Figure 12.3 Flow diagram to differentiate patient–prosthesis mismatch from obstruction in an aortic valve.

Table 12.6 Grading of patient–prosthesis mismatch by indexed effective orifice area (cm²/m²)[5]

	Moderate	Severe
BMI <30		
Aortic	0.66–0.85	≤0.65
Mitral	0.9–1.2	<0.9
BMI ≥30		
Aortic	0.56–0.70	≤0.55
Mitral	0.8–1.0	<0.8

- If there are no baseline or other earlier studies, Table 12.7 suggests when to suspect obstruction.
- Pressure half-time does not reflect orifice area in normally functioning prosthetic mitral valves, but it lengthens significantly when the valve becomes obstructed (Figure 12.4).

3. Is there regurgitation, and is it pathological?

If regurgitation is detected, it must be categorised as normal or pathological based on its origin and grade.

3.1 Origin of the jet

- How many jets, and are they through the valve (Figure 12.2), paraprosthetic, or both? Localisation can only be certain if the base or neck of the jet can be imaged in relation to the sewing ring.

Table 12.7 **When to suspect significant prosthetic valve obstruction with an isolated study**[1, 2]

Symptoms
Thickened or immobile cusps or occluder
Narrowed colour map across the valve
Measurements outside normal values (Appendix Tables A.8– A.10)
Aortic position: • V_{max} >4.0 m/s (see also Figure 12.3 if V_{max} >3.0 m/s) • Mean pressure difference >35 mmHg • EOA <0.8 cm² • Acceleration time >100 ms*
Mitral position: • Pressure half-time >200 ms and V_{max} >2.5 m/s • Mean gradient >10mmHg • DVI ($VTI_{mitral}/VTI_{subaortic}$) >2.5
Pulmonary position: • V_{max} >2.0 m/s for homograft or >3.0 m/s for any other valve type
Tricuspid position: • Pressure half-time >230 ms • Mean gradient >6 mmHg • V_{max} >1.6 m/s
Indirect signs: • Rise in TR V_{max} • Dilatation of RV (any valve, but especially pulmonary) • Dilatation or hypokinesis of LV (aortic)

* Acceleration time is the time from the onset to the peak of the transaortic CW signal.

- For a mechanical valve, the jets through the valve should match the typical pattern expected of the design (Figure 12.2).
- Regurgitation through the valve in bileaflet mechanical valves ('pivotal washing jets') begins close to the edge of the orifice and must not be mistaken for paraprosthetic jets.
- The site and extent of a paraprosthetic aortic jet can be described on the sewing ring as a clockface in the parasternal short-axis view.

3.2 Severity of regurgitation

- Normal regurgitation through a mechanical valve is usually low in momentum (relatively homogeneous colour), with an incomplete or very low-intensity continuous wave signal.
- For larger jets, use the same methods as for native regurgitation (see Chapters 8–10). Assessing the height of a jet relative to LVOT diameter may be difficult since paraprosthetic jets are often eccentric.

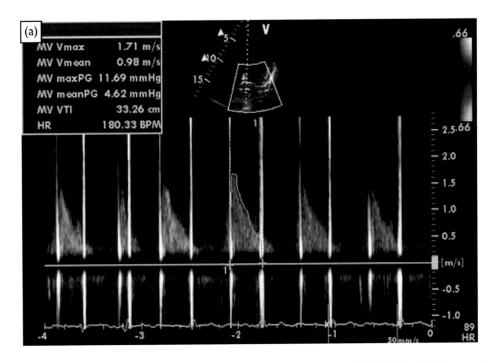

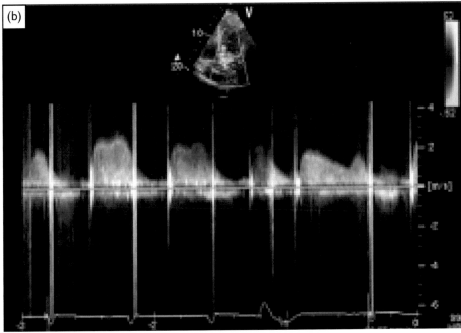

Figure 12.4 **Obstruction in a mitral prosthetic valve.** The transmitral Doppler signal is shown soon (a) after implantation with a pressure half-time 50 ms, and (b) after stopping warfarin when the patient was admitted with pulmonary oedema and a pressure half-time 350 ms.

- The circumference of the sewing ring occupied by the jet is another approximate guide. For a surgical valve in the aortic position, a jet occupying >20% of the circumference on TTE is likely severe. 3D TOE is required for the mitral position.
- TAVI may have multiple jets, and these may occur both through and around the valve. Quantification is often difficult using echocardiography. If accurate quantification is needed, consider CMR.
- Severe paraprosthetic MR may be obvious from:
  - A large region of flow convergence within the LV.
  - A broad neck.
  - A hyperdynamic LV.
  - A dense continuous wave signal, especially with early depressurisation (dagger shape).

4. Is there other disease?

- Assess all other valves, LV and RV function, and PA pressures.
- A hyperdynamic LV is a clue that there may be severe prosthetic aortic or mitral regurgitation.
- A rise in pulmonary artery pressure can be a sign of prosthetic mitral valve obstruction.

When is TOE indicated?

TTE and TOE are complementary, and TOE is rarely used without initial TTE (Table 12.8). Although TOE is usually necessary to image vegetations and posterior root abscesses, anterior root abscesses may be better seen on TTE.

Table 12.8 **Indications for TOE**

Endocarditis clinically likely
Obstruction suggested by TTE to: • Image leaflets   • Detect thrombus, pannus, or vegetations
To image leaflet opening to differentiate patient prosthesis mismatch from pathological obstruction in an aortic valve prosthetic
Haemolysis (small regurgitant jet often not detected on TTE)
Symptomatic patient and suboptimal TTE imaging
Paraprosthetic mitral regurgitation of uncertain severity
Thromboembolism despite therapeutic INR (to detect pannus or thrombus)

MISTAKES TO AVOID

- Mistaking normal regurgitant jets in bileaflet mechanical valves, which begin close to the edge of the orifice for paraprosthetic jets.
- Overdiagnosing obstruction with a single high V_{max}.
- Failing to use off-axis views to detect flow convergence and the neck of a paraprosthetic mitral regurgitant jet.
- Not responding to a hyperdynamic LV as an indirect sign of severe paraprosthetic aortic or mitral regurgitation.
- Not doing a TOE to look for a small paraprosthetic jet if there is clinically severe haemolysis.

CHECKLIST FOR ECHOCARDIOGRAPHY OF PROSTHETIC VALVES

1. Appearance of the valve.
2. V_{max}, mean gradient, and effective orifice area (aortic) and pressure half-time (mitral and tricuspid).
3. Presence, location, and grade of regurgitation.
4. If velocities and gradients high: Is there evidence of pathological obstruction? Is there patient prosthesis mismatch?
5. LV size and function.
6. RV size and function and pulmonary pressure.
7. Aorta:
   a. Size of ascending aorta.
   b. Evidence of coarctation if the valve prosthetic was for a bicuspid aortic valve.

References

1. Lancellotti P, Pibarot P, Chambers J, et al. Recommendations for the imaging assessment of prosthetic heart valves. A report from the European Association of Cardiovascular Imaging endorsed by the Chinese Society of Echocardiography. Europ Heart J CVI 2016;17(6):589–90.
2. Zoghbi WA, Chambers JB, Dumesnil JG, et al. American Society of Echocardiography recommendations for evaluation of prosthetic valves with two-dimensional and Doppler echocardiography. J Am Soc Echo 2009;22(9):975–1014.

3. Zamorano JL, Badano LP, Bruce C, et al. EAE/ASE Recommendations for the use of echocardiography in new transcatheter interventions for valvular heart disease. JASE 2011;24:937–65 and Europ Heart J 2011;32(17):2189–214.
4. Pibarot P, Hermann HC, Changfu W, et al. Standardized definition of bioprosthetic valve dysfunction following aortic or mitral valve replacement. J Am Coll Cardiol 2022;80(5):545–61.
5. Pibarot P & Dumesnil JG. Valve prosthesis-patient mismatch, 1978 to 2011: From original concept to compelling evidence. J Am Coll Cardiol 2012;60(13):1136–9.

Endocarditis

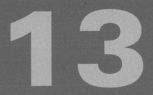

- Infective endocarditis is uncommon[1] but important because the mortality is up to 20%, and about 50% need inpatient cardiac surgery[2].
- Echocardiography is essential for:
  - Aiding the diagnosis when clinically suggested by contributing vegetations or local complications to the Duke criteria (Appendix Table A.7) as major criteria. TTE should not be done for fever alone.
  - Assessing the resulting valve regurgitation.
  - Planning surgery.

1. Is there a vegetation?

- This is typically a mass attached to the valve and moving with a different phase to the leaflet. However, there may sometimes be new thickening integral to the leaflet.
- It may be difficult to differentiate from other types of masses (e.g. calcific or myxomatous degeneration, a fibrin strand, or flail chord). This is a particular problem if TTE has been requested with a low clinical likelihood of endocarditis. Choose a descriptive term that will not lead to overdiagnosis of endocarditis (Table 13.1).
- Note the size and mobility of the vegetation. Highly mobile masses longer than 10 mm have a relatively high risk of embolisation and may affect the decision for and timing of surgery[3]. Vegetations longer than 15 mm are an indication for surgery in their own right.
- Vegetations usually occur on valves but also at the site of jet lesions or around the orifice of a VSD or on pacing leads.

2. Is there a local complication?

- A new paraprosthetic leak (dehiscence) is a reliable sign of replacement valve endocarditis, provided there is a baseline post-operative study showing no leak.
- Perforation, fistula.
- An abscess usually suggests that surgery will be necessary.
- TTE is good for showing anterior root abscesses (Figure 13.1); TOE better for posterior root abscesses.

149

DOI: 10.1201/9781003242789-13

Table 13.1 **Suggested terms for describing a mass**

• 'Typical of a vegetation'
• 'Consistent with a vegetation'
• 'Consistent but not diagnostic of a vegetation'
• 'Consistent with a vegetation but more in keeping with calcific degeneration'
• 'Most consistent with calcific degeneration'

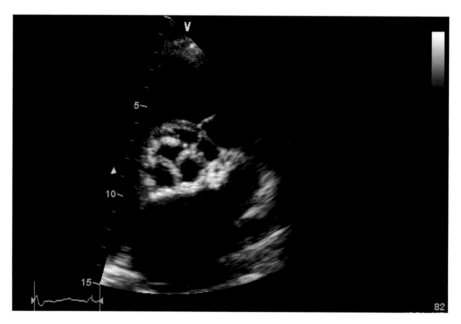

Figure 13.1 **Aortic abscess.** Parasternal short-axis view showing cavities between the pulmonary artery and aorta and in the anterior aorta. The aortic valve cusps are thickened because of endocarditis.

3. **Is there valve destruction?**
   - This may show as:
     - Disruption of the leaflet tissue with unusual patterns of movement, 'dog-legs,' or small flail segments (Figure 13.2).
     - A perforation.
     - New prolapse.
     - New or worsening regurgitation.

4. **Check the other valves**
   - Multiple valve involvement is particularly likely with invasive organisms, e.g. *Staphylococcus aureus*.
   - The jet of AR may impinge on the anterior mitral leaflet to seed a vegetation or cause local infection leading to an aneurysm or perforation.

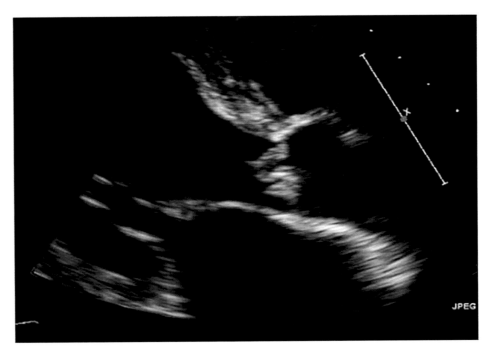

Figure 13.2 **Valve destruction.**

5. **Grade regurgitation**
    - This is as for regurgitation from any cause (Chapters 8–10).
    - The colour jet and spectral Doppler may be difficult to interpret because of artefact caused by the vibration of a vegetation, ruptured chord, or torn leaflet (Figure 13.3). A hyperdynamic LV is a clue to severe regurgitation.
    - The presence of severe regurgitation is an indication for surgery.

6. **Assess the LV**
    - Progressive systolic dilatation of the LV suggests the need for urgent surgery.
    - If there is acute severe AR, look for (Figure 8.7):
        - A transmitral E deceleration time <150 ms on pulsed Doppler.
        - Diastolic mitral regurgitation.
    - These are 'red flag' signs of a raised LV end-diastolic pressure and an indication for urgent or emergency surgery.
    - If you see these 'red flag' signs, immediately inform the clinician in charge of the case.

7. **Detect a predisposing abnormality**
    - About one-half of cases develop on previously normal valves. For the others, predisposing abnormalities are given in Table 13.2.
    - Pacemaker and implantable defibrillator endocarditis is increasingly common.

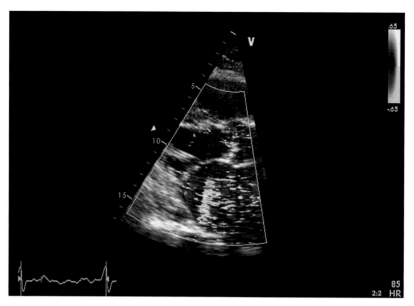

Figure 13.3 **Comb artefact.** This is caused by the vibration of a vegetation attached to the posterior mitral leaflet and leads to colour filling the left atrium and extending outside the heart.

 And here's an electronic link to a loop on the website or use
http://goo.gl/0kP3od

Table 13.2 **Predisposing abnormalities[1, 4]**

Prior endocarditis
Replacement or repaired heart valve
Native heart valve disease
Unrepaired cyanotic heart disease (or residual shunt)
Congenital disease repaired with a prosthetic valve
Hypertrophic cardiomyopathy
Implantable pacemaker or defibrillator

8. **TTE normal despite a clinical suspicion of endocarditis**

- This requires clinical discussion and depends on the clinical likelihood of endocarditis, how ill the patient is, and the quality of the TTE images.
- If the clinical likelihood is low or an alternative diagnosis emerges, further echocardiography is not indicated.
- If the clinical likelihood is moderate or high, choices include immediate TOE or a further TTE ± TOE after five to seven days[2].

Table 13.3 **Indications for TOE in endocarditis**

• Prosthetic valve, especially mechanical, if diagnosis not established
• Pacemaker or implantable defibrillator (pre- or intra-extraction procedure)
• Suspicion of abscess on transthoracic study or clinically (e.g. long PR interval)
• Normal or equivocal transthoracic study and moderate or high clinical suspicion of endocarditis

9. **When is TOE necessary?**
   - Established indications are given in Table 13.3.
   - TOE is commonly necessary if there is a prosthetic valve or pacemaker or defibrillator, because the yield of vegetations and complications is far higher than with TTE.
   - Guidelines[2] suggest a low threshold for requesting TOE even if the diagnosis has been established by TTE. The rationale is to refine the assessment of vegetation size and exclude abscesses. In clinical practice, TOE is not usually necessary if the results are not expected to change management (e.g. decision for surgery already made).

10. **Other imaging modalities**
   - Echocardiography, even with TOE, may fail to show evidence of endocarditis in replacement valves or infected pacing systems. This is partly because of shielding and partly because vegetations or local complication may not occur.
   - If the diagnosis remains clinically likely, **PET CT** should be considered.
   - A **CT** scan may be requested before cardiac surgery to avoid the need for invasive coronary angiography. CT may better define a complication like a para-aortic aneurysm or occasionally show complications not obvious on TTE and TOE.

Table 13.4 **Red flag signs on the echocardiogram in endocarditis**

Severe AR, especially with E deceleration time <150 ms and diastolic mitral regurgitation
Severe MR, especially if the LV is hyperdynamic (confirming severe MR) or hypodynamic (end-stage)
Abscess
Large (>15 mm), mobile vegetations
Rocking replacement valve

MISTAKES TO AVOID

- Using TTE as part of a fever screen, since it then has a very low yield and risks detecting 'innocent bystander' abnormalities (e.g. coincidental valve thickening).
- Reporting innocent bystander findings as vegetations.
- Missing progressive valve regurgitation as a sign of endocarditis.
- Overusing TOE when it will not change management.
- Assuming that the absence of a vegetation refutes the diagnosis.
- Not alerting the clinician in charge of the case to positive findings and particularly red flag signs (Table 13.4).

CHECKLIST REPORT IN ENDOCARDITIS

1. Is there a vegetation? How long and how mobile?
2. Is there a local complication or evidence of valve destruction?
3. Grade of regurgitation?
4. Presence and severity of predisposing disease (e.g. valve stenosis or VSD).
5. LV dimensions and function (or RV for tricuspid valve endocarditis).
6. Is there a mitral E deceleration time <150 ms or diastolic MR as evidence of high LV filling pressures?
7. Have you informed the clinician in charge of the case if there is evidence of endocarditis, severe valve regurgitation, and/or a restrictive LV filling pattern?

References

1. Thornhill M, Jones S, Prendergast B, et al. Quantifying infective endocarditis risk in patients with predisposing cardiac conditions. Europ Heart J 2018;39(7):586–95.
2. Habib G, Lancellotti P, Antunes MJ, et al. 2015 ESC Guidelines for the management of infective endocarditis. Europ Heart J 2015;36(44):3075–128.
3. Thuny F, Disalvo G, Belliard O, Avierinos JF, Pergola V, Rosenberg V, et al. Risk of embolism and death in infective endocarditis: Prognostic value of echocardiography: A prospective multicenter study. Circulation 2005;112(1):69–75.
4. Verheugt CL, Uiterwaal CSPM, van der Velde ET, et al. Turning 18 with congenital heart disease: Prediction of infective endocarditis based on a very large population. Eur Heart J 2011;32(15):1926–34.

The Heart Valve Clinic | 14

A heart valve clinic is the best practice method of assessing new patients with valve disease and following them during 'watchful waiting'[1, 2].

- The arrangements needed beyond a normal TTE list[3] are given in Box 14.1.
- A guide to setting up a new clinic is available on the British Heart Valve Society website[3].
- The visit comprises a clinical assessment with or without TTE.
- The usual frequency of follow-up is given in Table 14.1. This can be modified for individuals according to clinical need or the exigencies of COVID-19[3], including virtual assessment as appropriate.
- The components of the TTE can be individualised. A comprehensive study is needed on the first visit, but thereafter, the cardiologist or clinical scientist can sometimes focus the study. For example, it is not necessary to study the pulmonary valve repeatedly if known to be normal. Points to cover in the history are given in Box 14.2.

Box 14.1 Organisational requirements for a valve clinic

- Experienced staff with specialist valve competencies.
- Agree types of patients to be seen and link with staff, for example, nurse to see cases post-intervention not requiring TTE, senior physiologist or clinical scientist to see patients with asymptomatic moderate and severe native valve disease, cardiologist for new and complex patients.
- Multidisciplinary meetings for difficult decisions and quality assurance.
- Referral links to: cardiac surgery and valve interventional services, other cardiac services (e.g. heart failure and electrophysiology), and non-cardiac services (e.g. dental, elderly care).
- Links to other tests, e.g., BNP, exercise testing, stress echo, TOE, CMR, CT, lung function.
- Inward referral, e.g., alerts in echocardiography lab, murmur clinic[4], links to open-access or community echocardiography services.
- Agreed set of criteria for referral from nurse or physiologist to the cardiologist (Figure 14.1).
- One-stop echocardiography.
- 'Hotline' for GPs and patients to report new symptoms.
- Patient information resources[4, 5].

DOI: 10.1201/9781003242789-14

155

Sonographer & Nurse led Clinics: Alerts & Frequency of Visit

Mitral Stenosis

Severe: every 6 months (ETT annually)
Moderate: every 1-2 years
Mild: every 2 years

Echocardiographic alerts:
- New PA hypertension or rise in PA systolic pressure towards 50 mmHg
- RV dysfunction

Other alerts:
- Symptoms
- INR > 4.0 or < 1.5 in last 6 months
- New atrial fibrillation
- TIA or stroke
- Patient request
- Suggestion of endocarditis

Mitral Regurgitation

Severe: every 6 months + annual ETT
Moderate: every 1-2 years
Mild: not followed

Echocardiographic alerts:
- LVSD approaching 40 mm
- LV EF approaching 60%
- PA systolic pressure approaching 50mmHg

Other alerts:
- Symptoms
- New arrhythmia
- Patient request
- Suggestion of endocarditis

Aortic Stenosis

V max >4.0 m/s or EOA < 1.0cm^2	every 6 months + consider annual ETT
V max 3.5 – 4.0 m/s + AV Calcium	every 6 months
V max 3.0 – 4.0 m/s or EOI 1.0 – 1.5cm^2	every year + ETT at baseline, when becomes severe, and consider every year after this if early surgery clinically appropriate
V max 2.5 – 3.0 m/s	every 3 years

Echocardiographic Alerts
- Any reduction in LV ejection fraction
- EOI $\leq$0.6cm^2
- V max $\geq$5.0m/s
- Rapid progression of V max > 0.3 m/s per year
- New diastolic dysfunction (pseudonormal or restrictive)
- Aortic root dilated to 45 mm (Marfan's), 55 mm (other)

Other Alerts
- Spontaneous symptoms
- New arrhythmia
- Patient request
- Suggestion of endocarditis

Aortic Regurgitation

Severe: every 6 months or every 3 months at request of cardiologist if LV significantly dilated (consider ETT annually)
Moderate: every 1-2 years
Mild: not unless aortic root dilated

Echocardiographic alerts:
- LVSD approaching 50 mm or LVDD 70 mm
- LVSD change (>5mm from previous study) or volume increase since last study
- LVEF approaching 50%

Other alerts:
- Spontaneous symptoms
- New arrhythmia
- Patient request
- Suggestion of endocarditis

Pulmonary Stenosis

Severe: every year
Moderate: every 1-2 years
Mild: no follow up unless indicated

Echocardiographic alerts:
- New RV dilation
- Velocity > 3.5 m/s

Other alerts:
- Spontaneous symptoms
- New arrhythmia
- Suggestion of endocarditis
- Patient request

Tricuspid / Pulmonary Regurgitation

Severe: every 6 months
Moderate: every 1-2 years

Echocardiographic alerts:
- Progressive RV dilatation
- New RV hypokinesis

Other alerts:
- Spontaneous symptoms
- New arrhythmia
- Suggestion of endocarditis
- Patient request

Figure 14.1 Suggested echocardiographic and clinical alerts for referral from nurse- or physiologist-led clinics to the cardiologist.

SOUTH LONDON
CARDIAC NETWORK **NHS**

Mitral & Tricuspid Valve Repair

– Echo at 12 months –
If repair, competent, continue clinical surveillance annually in nurse-led clinic.

If repair impaired, continue echo surveillance per native dysfunction.

Echocardiographic alerts:
- Worsening regurgitation – see MR/TR sections
- Systolic anterior motion

Other alerts:
- Spontaneous symptoms
- New arrhythmia
- Patient request
- Suggestion of endocarditis

Aortic Root Dilatation

Marfan: annually unless dilated to > 40 mm, then every 6 months
Non-Marfan: annually
Bicuspid: annually

Echocardiographic alerts:
- Marfan 45 mm or change > 3 mm in one year
- Bicuspid valve 55 mm or change > 3 mm in one year
- Non-Marfan 55 mm or change > 3 mm in one year
- Worsening AR

Other alerts:
- Chest pain, dysphagia or change in voice
- New arrhythmia
- Patient request
- Suggestion of endocarditis

Post-Endocarditis (non-operated)

Echocardiogram at 1, 3, and 6 months
Then according to residual pathology

Biscuspid Valve (no AS/AR)

Every 3 years

Replacement Heart Valves

Every valve once postoperatively if not performed before discharge

Mechanical valves annually only if there is any of the following:
- Associated root dilatation (see specific guide)
- LV dilatation
- More than mild paraprosthetic regurgitation
- More than moderate TR

New designs of biological aortic valve every year after 5 years (e.g. Trifecta)

Established aortic biological designs every year after 10 years

Biological mitral valves every year after 5 years

Ross procedures every year

AVR native root monitoring (previous bicuspid AV)
(Dimensions on post-op echo)

<40 mm	No routine surveillance
40 – 45 mm	Echo at 5 yearly then review
>45 mm	Annual echo

AVR with Aortic Root Replacement (Marfans/Ehlers Danlos)
Per valve type above
2 yearly CMR or CT scanning (renal bloods needed prior to scan)

Echocardiographic alerts:
- New or worsening regurgitation
- Obstruction – reduction of EOA by 25%
- Change in LV or systolic function (or RV for right-sided valves)

Other alerts:
- Exertional symptoms
- TIA
- INR > 4.0 or <2.0 during last 6 months
- New arrhythmia
- Patient request
- Suggestion of endocarditis

Figure 14.1 (Continued)

Table 14.1 **Usual frequency of TTE (clinical) follow-up*6, 7**

	Mild	Moderate	Severe
Aortic regurgitation	–	2 y (1 yr)	6–12/12 (6/12)*
Aortic stenosis	Young pts 2–3 yr (2–3 yr)	1 yr (1 yr)	6/12 (6/12)*
Primary mitral regurgitation	3–5 yr (3–5 yr) (with mitral prolapse; otherwise, not needed)	1–2 yrs (1yr)	6/12 (6/12)*
Mitral stenosis	–	2–3 yr (2–3 yr)	1 yr (1 yr)
Dilated aorta	1 yr (1 yr) (may need MRI or CT)		
Bicuspid aortic valve	3–5 yr (with no AR or AS and no aortic dilatation)		
Repaired mitral valve	Baseline and 1 yr, then according to any residual MR		

* More frequently if close to thresholds for surgery.

Box 14.2 Points to cover in the routine annual follow-up

Includes native and post-repair or replacement surgery.

History
- New symptoms? Change in exercise capacity? Slowing down?
- Psychological or cognitive issues, including understanding of the condition.
- What to look out for (TIA, bleeding, fever, breathlessness).
- Management of other conditions (e.g. COPD).
- Medication check.

Examination
- New AF? Blood pressure?
- Progression of valve disease?
- Evidence of heart failure?
- Post-surgery scar problems: keloid, pain, wire protruding.

Anticoagulation
- INR control: Stable? Frequency of testing? Diet if INR variable? Bleeding? Home testing?

- Correct INR range?
- Could a NOAC be indicated (valve disease other than mechanical prosthesis or mitral stenosis)?
- When can warfarin stop after surgery?
- Perioperative anticoagulant bridging.
- Contraception and pregnancy planning advice.

Endocarditis advice

- Dental surveillance and antibiotic prophylaxis.
- Other advice (e.g. tattoo, piercing).
- What symptoms to look out for.

Lifestyle advice

- Smoking cessation.
- Weight loss.
- Exercise.

Table 14.2 **Suggested start time for routine annual TTE in normally functioning prosthetic valves**[8]

Mechanical		
Not needed in the absence of another indication (e.g. dilated aorta)		
Biological		
Onset of routine TTE	**Risk of early failure**	**Valve types**
From implantation	High or unknown	TAVI New designs
After 5 years from implantation	Higher	Mitral or tricuspid position Aortic position implanted at age <50 or with risk factors: diabetes, hypertension, renal failure
After 10 years from implantation	Lower	Designs with good durability data (e.g. Hancock II, Perimount)

References

1. Lancellotti P, Rosenhek R, Pibarot P, et al. Heart valve clinics: Organisation, structure and experiences. Eur Heart J 2013;34(21):1597–606.
2. Chambers JB. Valve clinic: Why, who and how? Education in Heart. Heart 2019;105:1913–20.
3. BHVS link to guide to setting up a valve clinic. https://bhvs.org/bhvs-set-up-valve-clinic/
4. BHVS link to patient information leaflets. https://bhvs.org/patient-information/
5. BHVS link to patient book. https://bhvs.org/product/patient-book/
6. Vahanian A, Beyersdorf F, Praz F, et al. 2021 ESC/EACTS Guidelines for the management of valvular heart disease. Eur Heart J 2022;43(7):561–632.
7. Otto CM, Nishimura RA, Bonow RO, et al. 2020 ACC/AHA Guideline for the management of patients with valvular heart disease: A report of the American College of Cardiology/American Heart Association Joint Committee on Clinical Practice Guidelines. Circulation 2021;143(5):e72–227.
8. Chambers J, Briffa N, Garbi M & Steed RV. Echocardiography in replacement heart valves. Echo Research Pract 2019. doi.org/10.1530/ERP-18–0079.

The Aorta and Dissection

15

The Aorta

1. Where to measure

- The diameter of the sinus, sinotubular junction, and ascending thoracic aorta is measured in the parasternal long-axis view in the minimum standard study (Chapter 1).
- Upper limits of normal values are given in Figure 15.1.
- Diameters at other levels (arch, descending thoracic, and abdominal aorta) require multiple views and should be measured if there is a high likelihood of dilatation:
  - Dilatation of the root or ascending aorta on the initial views
  - Significant aortic valve disease (stenosis or regurgitation)
  - Bicuspid aortic valve
  - Congenital and genetic syndromes associated with aortic dilatation, for example, Marfan syndrome (Table 15.1)
- A short-axis view at the level of the sinus of Valsalva should be recorded since this may show asymmetric dilatation of the sinuses. Measure from the apex of the sinus to the aorta between the sinuses diametrically opposite.
- CT or MRI are indicated if the ascending aorta is not well seen on TTE and there is a high likelihood of dilatation.

2. How to measure

- There is no published consensus on the method for measuring aortic dimensions, but most echocardiography departments do the following (Figure 15.2):
  - 2D rather than M-mode measured perpendicular to the long-axis.
  - 'Inner edge to inner edge' rather than 'leading edge to leading edge'.
  - Most guidelines suggest measurement of the annulus in mid-systole but the rest of the aorta at end-diastole. In practice, the timing of the clearest image may not be exact, and it is then reasonable to measure in systole[3].
- Individual departments should agree on a standard. When comparing serial data, it is important to assess measurements made in an equivalent manner and at comparable points in the cardiac cycle. This may require reanalysis of previous data using the current convention, where required.

DOI: 10.1201/9781003242789-15

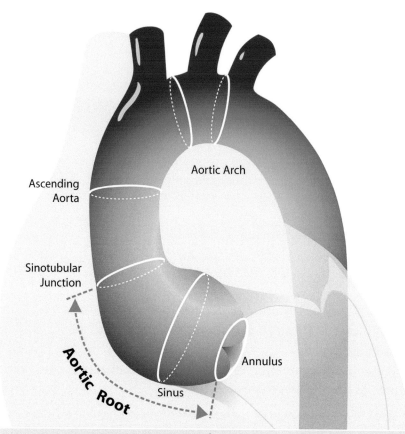

Upper limit of normal for aortic root diameters according to age and sex			
Male	**<40 yrs**	**30-59 yrs**	**≥60 yrs**
Annulus (mm)	24.8	24.9	25.8
Sinus of Valsava (mm)	37.2	39.2	39.3
Sinotubular Junction (mm)	32.4	35.7	37.3
Ascending aorta (mm)	34.2	37.5	41.4
Female	**<40 yrs**	**30-59 yrs**	**≥60 yrs**
Annulus (mm)	22.5	22.0	21.3
Sinus of Valsava (mm)	33.4	33.3	33.5
Sinotubular Junction (mm)	30.5	31.5	32.9
Ascending aorta (mm)	31.6	33.6	38.6

Figure 15.1 Levels and normal values for measuring the diameter of the aorta. Upper limits are calculated from the NORRE dataset[1, 2] as mean +2 standard deviations.

Table 15.1 **Causes of aortic dilatation**

Atherosclerosis
Congenital/genetic causes: Bicuspid aortic valve, familial thoracic aortic aneurysm, Marfan syndrome, Ehlers–Danlos type IV, Loeys–Dietz, Turner's syndrome, autosomal dominant polycystic kidney disease
Infections: Mycotic aortitis, syphilis, *Staphylococcus aureus* aortitis
Inflammatory causes: Takayasu arteritis, giant cell arteritis, Behcet's arteritis, rheumatoid arthritis, ankylosing spondylitis
Trauma: Cardiac catheterization or deceleration injury or, rarely late, after prior dissection

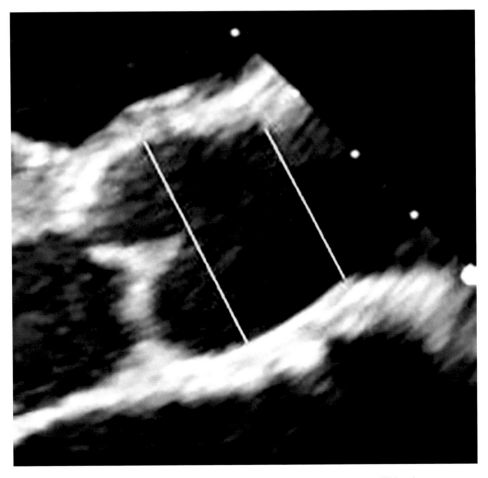

Figure 15.2 **Method of measuring the aortic diameter.** This shows a representative parasternal long-axis view of the aorta for measuring diameters at the sinus of Valsalva, sinotubular junction, and ascending aorta in diastole. The annulus is measured in systole.

3. Is the aorta dilated?

- Upper limits of normal using the large NORRE dataset are given in Figure 15.1[1, 2].
- Where the measurement is borderline:
    - If the patient is at an extreme of body size, index to height (Appendix Figures A.1 and A.2 for nomograms).
    - Repeating the measurement after a delay of six or so months is an option to confirm stability[4].

- The Z score is the number of standard deviations between the observed measurement and the mean expected using formulae derived from age, sex, and either height or BSA[5]. This is useful in growing children.
- Commonly used age-independent thresholds for dilatation are:
    - Ascending aorta >41 mm (>21mm/m^2)
    - Arch >36 mm
    - Descending aorta >35 mm (>16 mm/m^2)
    - Abdominal aorta >30 mm

- A difference in proportion can be used to diagnose dilatation, for example, an ascending/descending thoracic aortic diameter >1.5. The diameter of the ascending aorta and sinotubular junction should be similar and both slightly larger than the annulus.
- The shape may give a guide to the presence of dilatation[6] and the cause:
    - Marfan syndrome: typically 'pear-shaped' annuloaortic ectasia.
    - Bicuspid valve: ascending aorta more than sinus.
    - Atherosclerosis (degenerative): sinus and ascending aorta.

- A coronary sinus aneurysm can be missed if short-axis views are not examined (Table 15.3). Use colour flow and spectral Doppler to look for fenestrations. Coronary sinus rupture is a cause of LV volume overload.

4. Cut points for surgery

- If thresholds for surgery are close, it is usual to confirm dimensions using orthogonal planes provided by CT or CMR.
- Despite the aortic size being related to body habitus, minimum thresholds for considering referral for surgery are based on absolute diameters (Table 15.3) other than for people with height-limiting syndromes. The decision for surgery

Table 15.2 **Coronary sinus aneurysm**

Sinus involved	Site of extension
Right	RV outflow tract
Left	Left atrium
Non-coronary	Right atrium

Table 15.3 Guideline thresholds for prophylactic intervention in thoracic aortic aneurysm[7, 8]

	Guideline diameter for considering intervention
Ascending aorta or sinus of Valsalva	
No associated conditions	≥50 mm Or ≥45 mm with risk factors* or at time of aortic valve surgery or prior to pregnancy
Bicuspid aortic valve	≥55 mm Or ≥50 mm with risk factors* or prior to pregnancy Or ≥45 mm if aortic valve surgery planned
Marfan syndrome	≥50 mm (root) ≥45 mm (root) with risk factors* or prior to pregnancy Cross-sectional root area:height ratio ≥10
Turner syndrome	≥25 mm/m^2 prior to pregnancy
Loeys–Dietz syndrome (or TGFBR1 or 2 mutation)	Individualise Or ≥45 mm prior to pregnancy
Ehlers–Danlos syndrome	No specific threshold
Familial thoracic aortic aneurysm	No specific threshold
Aortic arch	
None	≥55 mm
Descending thoracic aorta	
Suitable for stent graft	≥55 mm
Needs open surgery	≥60 mm

* Risk factors: High rate of increase (≥5 mm/yr if no associated conditions, otherwise ≥3 mm/yr), family history of dissection, uncontrolled hypertension, coarctation.

takes account of many clinical factors (e.g. coronary disease, valve disease) and must be individualised.

5. Other features

- **Is the aortic wall thickened** (≥5 mm)?
- **Is there atherosclerosis?** This is usually best seen by TOE. However, on good-quality TTE, atheroma may be seen in the ascending aorta and arch.
- **Is there significant calcification in the aorta?** Severe calcification may affect the feasibility of coronary bypass and valve surgery.
- **How much aortic regurgitation** (page 94)?

- **Has the aortic diameter changed from previous studies?** A significant rate of increase is taken as ≥5 mm/year if there are no associated conditions but otherwise ≥3 mm/year[9]. Check by comparing the images that the measurements were taken at the same level and in the same part of the cycle.

- **How long is the abnormal part of the aorta?** If the ascending aorta is dilated, check whether the arch and descending thoracic aorta are normal. This may require imaging using CT or MRI if TTE image quality is not adequate.

- **Check for coarctation** in all subjects, particularly if there is a bicuspid aortic valve, unexplained aortic dilatation, or hypertension in a young adult.

- **Is there mitral or tricuspid prolapse?** This is relevant in patients with Marfan or Ehlers–Danlos syndromes.

- **Is there coexistent pulmonary artery dilatation** (Table 10.7)? This may be seen in Marfan syndrome and, to a lesser degree, with a bicuspid aortic valve.

- **Consider measuring the descending thoracic and abdominal aorta.** Use all views. This should be done in:
  - Marfan and Ehlers–Danlos syndromes
  - Dissection
  - Dilatation of the aortic arch
  - Dilatation of the descending aorta shown on initial parasternal long-axis views

Dissection and Acute Aortic Syndromes

Acute aortic syndrome is characterised by instantaneous-onset chest pain. There is often an underlying predisposition (e.g. Marfan syndrome, known aortic valve, or aortic disease). There may be suggestive clinical findings (asymmetric pulses or blood pressure).

- The main cause is dissection, which may involve the ascending aorta (Stanford type A) or affect the descending aorta alone (Stanford type B) (Figure 15.3).

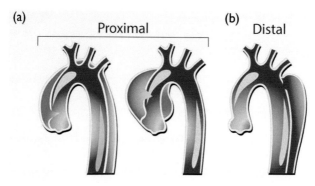

(a) Proximal   (b) Distal

Figure 15.3 Classification of dissections. Type A dissections involve the ascending aorta. Type B dissections involve only the descending thoracic aorta.

- TTE has 80% sensitivity for type A and 50% for type B dissections, potentially allowing the initial diagnosis to be made in the emergency room.
- If the initial TTE is non-diagnostic, CT or TOE are indicated to detect a dissection or the other causes of acute aortic syndrome: intramural haematoma (20%), penetrating atherosclerotic ulcer (5%), aortic pseudoaneurysms, and contained or free rupture (usually after trauma or surgery).

1. **Is there a dissection flap?**
    - An intraluminal flap is the hallmark of dissection. Blooming from calcium deposits or reverberation artefact can sometimes cause confusion. Factors suggesting artefact:
        - Fixed relationship with a heavy reflector, for example, anterior aortic wall.
        - No movement at a phase different from the aorta.
        - Only apparent in certain views.
        - 'Pseudoflap' extends outside the aorta.
        - The 'pseudoflap' has no effect on colour Doppler (a real flap would divide colour onto true and false lumens, or there would be increased velocities through entry tears).
    - Echocardiography has several goals in the assessment of aortic dissection (Table 15.4).
    - Echocardiographic findings can aid the differentiation between true and false lumens (Table 15.5).
    - If there is a high clinical suspicion for aortic dissection but the TTE appears normal:
        - Check all views, including suprasternal and right intercostal.
        - Consider intramural haematoma. Check for thickening of the aortic wall (>5 mm).
        - Consider CT or, occasionally, TOE according to availability.

2. **What is the maximum aortic diameter?**
    Dissection is unlikely in an aorta of normal diameter.

3. **How much aortic regurgitation?**
    If present, determine its severity (Chapter 8). Possible mechanisms are given in Table 15.6, but the decision for aortic valve replacement is made at surgery guided by TOE.

4. **Is there pericardial fluid?**
    This suggests rupture into the pericardial sac, which is a common cause of death in acute dissection. It may suggest the diagnosis even if a flap cannot be imaged.

Table 15.4 **Role of echocardiography in diagnosing aortic dissection and assessing its complications***

Diagnostic goal	Echocardiographic definition
Identify presence of a dissection flap.	A flap that divides two lumens.
Define extension of the aortic dissection.	Proximal and distal extent of the flap, true and false lumens (Table 15.5).
Localise entry tear.	Disruption of the flap with flow through the site of the tear.
Thrombosis of the false lumen.	Mass inside the false lumen.
Presence, severity, and mechanism of aortic regurgitation.	See Table 15.6 for mechanisms and Chapter 8 for grading severity.
Coronary involvement.	New regional wall motion abnormality in RCA territory occasionally with involvement of the flap with the RCA ostium. Dissection does not cause new anterior infarcts.
Aortic branch involvement.	Flap invagination into aortic branches.
Detect pericardial and/or pleural effusions.	Echo-free pericardial/pleural space (Chapter 17).

* All features are better seen by TOE than TTE, but TTE is better at showing the distal extent of the dissection in the abdominal aorta, LV wall motion, and assessing valve regurgitation.

Table 15.5 **Differentiating between the true and false lumen[10]**

	True lumen	False lumen
Size	Usually false larger than true	
Pulsation	Systolic expansion	Systolic compression
Flow direction	Normal systolic antegrade flow	Reduced systolic antegrade flow or delayed, absent, or reversed flow
Communication flow	From true to false lumen in systole	

Table 15.6 **Mechanisms of aortic regurgitation seen in aortic dissection[10]**

Dilatation of the sinus of Valsalva, sinotubular junction, or aortic annulus
Rupture of the annular support and a tear at the insertion point of a valve leaflet
Intramural haematoma distorting the valve
Prolapse of the intima into the LV outflow tract
Previous aortic valve disease

5. LV function

- Severe impairment of LV function on TTE can guide the decision towards conservative management, especially in dissections involving only the descending thoracic aorta.
- An inferior wall motion abnormality may occur as a result of ascending aortic dissection involving the right coronary artery.

MISTAKES TO AVOID

- Making oblique measurements of the aortic diameter, particularly in off-axis views.
- Overdiagnosis of dissection from a reverberation artefact.
- Exclusion of dissection with TTE alone. TTE is a good screening procedure, but a negative result is not definitive and should be supplemented with CT or TOE.
- Failing to image the ascending aorta when clinically necessary.
- Monitoring aortic size using TTE alone if image quality is not adequate.

CHECKLIST REPORT FOR THE AORTA

1. Diameter at each level. Re-measure and compare serial studies. Have any measurements changed?
2. Check for abnormalities associated with a dilated aorta, for example, coarctation, bicuspid aortic valve.
3. Is there associated AR? Grade?
4. If there is suspected dissection: Is there a flap? Is there abnormal LV wall motion? Is there a pericardial effusion?

References

1. Kou S, Caballero L, Dulgheru R, et al. Echocardiographic reference ranges for normal cardiac chamber size: Results from the NORRE study. Eur Heart J Cardiovasc Imaging 2014;15(6):680–90.
2. Saura D, Dulgheru R, Caballero L, et al. Two-dimensional transthoracic echocardiographic normal reference ranges for proximal aorta dimensions: Results from the EACVI NORRE study. Eur Heart J CVI 2017;18(2):167–79.
3. Lang RM, Badano LP, Mor-Avi V, et al. Recommendations for cardiac chamber quantification by echocardiography in adults: An update from the American Society

of Echocardiography and the European Association of Cardiovascular Imaging. J Am Soc Echocardiogr 2015;28(1):1–39.

4. Zafar MA, Li Y, Rizzo JA, et al. Height alone, rather than body surface area, suffices for risk estimation in ascending aortic aneurysm. J Thorac Cardiovasc Surg 2018;155(5):1938–50.

5. Devereux RB, de Simone G, Arnett DK, et al. Normal limits in relation to age, body size and gender of two-dimensional echocardiographic aortic root dimensions in persons ≥15 years of age. Am J Cardiol 2012;110(8):1189–94.

6. Detaint D, Michelena HI, Nkomo VVT, et al. Aortic dilatation patterns and rates in adults with bicuspid aortic valves. Heart 2014;100(2):126–34.

7. Isselbacher EM, Preventza O, Black JH, et al. ACC/AHA Guideline for the diagnosis and management of aortic disease. J Am Coll Cardiol 2022;80(24):e223–e393.

8. Erbel R, Aboyans V, Boileau C, et al. 2014 ESC Guidelines on the diagnosis and treatment of aortic diseases: Document covering acute and chronic aortic diseases of the thoracic and abdominal aorta of the adult. Eur Heart J 2014;35(41):2873–926.

9. Evangelista A, Flachskampf FA, Erbel R, et al. Echocardiography in aortic diseases: EAE Recommendations for clinical practice. Eur J Echocardiogr. 2010;11(8):645–58.

10. Goldstein SA, Evangelista A, Abbara S, et al. Multimodality imaging of diseases of the thoracic aorta in adults. J Am Soc Echocardiogr 2015;28(2):119–82.

Adult Congenital Heart Disease

16

- Patients with congenital disease should be cared for at specialist centres, but they may still present as an emergency or be followed at a non-specialist centre with uncorrected simple lesions, or after intervention[1].
- Examples of echocardiographic abnormalities found in congenital syndromes are given in Table 16.1.
- A first diagnosis of a simple, or occasionally, a more complex, lesion may still be made in a general echocardiography laboratory. This chapter describes:
  - Simple defects.
  - A sequential segmental approach to an unexpected complex case.
  - The appearances after intervention.
- Patients with congenital disease may be admitted acutely because of cardiac or other disease. Advice should be sought from a regional centre, but findings of immediate concern include:
  - Poorly functioning LV or RV.
  - Severe valve obstruction or regurgitation.
  - Evidence of endocarditis (the risk is 20 times higher than for the general population, except for those with isolated pulmonary stenosis or ASD)[2].
  - Atrial arrhythmia, because of the risk of decompensation, especially in a Fontan circulation or with a single ventricle.

Simple Defects

1. **Atrial septal defect (ASD)**
   - This is the most common congenital defect found in adult practice (Table 16.2).
   - Suspect an ASD if the RV is dilated. Another cause of RV dilatation is partial anomalous pulmonary veins.
   - **Describe the position** (Figure 16.1):
     - **Secundum** (80%)—approximately in the centre of the septum. May be elliptical or round and can contain multiple fenestrations.
     - **Primum** (15%)—next to the atrioventricular valves (Table 16.3).
     - **Superior sinus venosus** (5%)—may be difficult to image transthoracically; CMR or TOE usually needed.

DOI: 10.1201/9781003242789-16

Table 16.1 **Echocardiographic abnormalities in congenital syndromes**

	Typical	Less common
Noonan	Dysplastic valvar pulmonary stenosis, HCM	ASD, VSD, branch PS, tetralogy of Fallot
Turner	Bic AV, aortic stenosis, coarctation, dilated aorta with risk of aortic dissection	Hypoplastic left heart
Williams	Supravalvar AS, coarctation	PA and branch stenosis
LEOPARD	Valvar PS, HCM	
DiGeorge	Tetralogy of Fallot, VSD, truncus arteriosus	Interrupted arch, aortic arch abnormalities
Klinefelter	PDA, ASD, MV prolapse	
Allagile	Branch PS, tetralogy of Fallot	VSD, ASD, AS, coarctation
Keutel	Branch PS	
Congenital rubella	Persistent duct, branch PS, coarctation	
Fetal alcohol	VSD, ASD	
Neurofibromatosis	Coarctation	
Loeys–Dietz	Aortic dilatation	Bicuspid aortic valve, persistent duct, ASD

- **Inferior sinus venosus** (<1%).
- **Coronary sinus defect** (unroofed coronary sinus) is not a true ASD but permits a left-to-right shunt from the LA via the coronary sinus to the RA.
- TTE has limited use in the assessment of anomalous pulmonary venous connections in adults with ASD[3, 4]. CMR is usually necessary.
- **Shunt direction?** In adult practice, this will be predominantly left to right, but if pulmonary vascular resistance is increased, flow may be bidirectional or right to left. Optimise the colour scale settings to 25–40 cm/s. For the detection of bidirectional shunting, use PW in addition to colour Doppler.
- **Estimate the anatomical and physiological size of the defect:**
  - RV dilatation (RV larger than LV in an apical 4-chamber view) implies a haemodynamically significant shunt and is an indication for closure.
  - The size can be measured approximately by callipers on 2D or 3D TTE without colour. Use 3D for an en-face view of the ASD.
  - ASD defects ≥10 mm in diameter, or defects that occupy >1/3 of the length of the total interatrial septum are usually significant and may require closure.

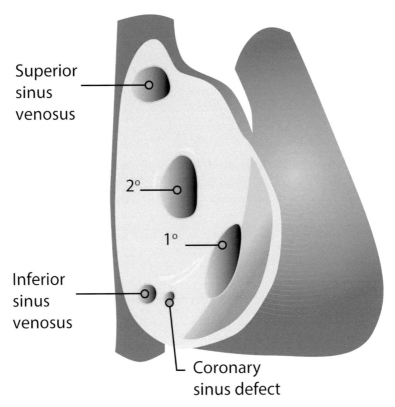

Superior
sinus
venosus

2°

1°

Inferior
sinus
venosus

Coronary
sinus defect

Figure 16.1 **Position of ASD.** 1° is a primum defect, and 2° is a secundum defect.

- The number of defects in the atrial septum should be quantified if multiple (fenestrated ASD defect).
- The estimated shunt (Qp/Qs) (see page 242) may aid the initial diagnosis and help determine whether closure is still indicated if there is pulmonary hypertension.
- 3D TTE refines assessment of the size, shape, and rims of the ASD and its proximity to the surrounding cardiac structures.
- Describe RV size and function (Chapter 4).
- Estimate pulmonary artery pressure (Chapter 5).
- The systolic pressure may be elevated because of high right-sided flow.
- If pulmonary resistance is not significantly raised, the diastolic pressure is normal or low.
- Usually, if the PA systolic pressure is >50% systemic pressure, it is advisable to measure PA pressures and resistance invasively before considering closure.
- **Describe LV size and function** (Chapter 2). LV function may decompensate after ASD closure.

Table 16.2 Checklist in ASD

Position (secundum, primum, sinus venosus)
Anatomical characteristics—size, shape, rims (including 3D TTE when available)
Aneurysmal atrial septum +/– prominent Eustachian valve or Chiari network
Number of defects
Direction of shunt (left to right, bidirectional, right to left)
Shunt size (Qp/Qs >1.5 indicates significant shunting)
RV size and function
PA pressure
LV size and function (may decompensate after ASD closure)
Other congenital or acquired defects?

Table 16.3 Features of a 'primum' ASD (part of the spectrum of atrioventricular septal defect)

Defect adjacent to the atrioventricular valves
Common atrioventricular valve rather than separate tricuspid and mitral valves Lack of offset between left- and right-sided atrioventricular valve Left atrioventricular valve appears 'cleft' or trileaflet
Long LV outflow tract caused by an offset between aortic valve and 'mitral valve' (normally the non-coronary aortic cusp is continuous with the base of the anterior mitral leaflet)
May be associated with a VSD

- If there is a primum defect (Table 16.3), look for a ventricular inlet defect and assess the atrioventricular valves.
- TOE is usually indicated before device closure (Table 16.4) and TTE afterwards.

- It is possible to mistake flow from the superior vena cava for flow across an ASD. Take multiple views. If there is still doubt, consider:
  - Saline contrast injection, which may make the ASD obvious as a void.
  - Pulsed Doppler on the right atrial side of the septum. ASD flow has a peak in late diastole and systole. For the superior vena cava, the peaks are earlier.
  - Shunt calculation (Appendix, page 242).
  - CMR or TOE, occasionally CT, or Intracardiac Echocardiography, if available.

2. **Ventricular septal defect** (Table 16.5)
   - In adults, a VSD may be newly diagnosed or unoperated as a child (either because it was too small or there was Eisenmenger syndrome).

Table 16.4 **TOE assessment before secundum ASD device closure**

How many defects or fenestrations?	
Total septal length	
Aneurysmal atrial septum?	
Prominent Eustachian valve?	
Diameters of defect (2D and 3D + colour flow Doppler)	
Rim distances to:	Aorta (a margin is not necessary when a septal occluder device is used)
	IVC and SVC
	Atrioventricular valves
Check correct drainage of pulmonary veins	
Other defects, especially cleft mitral valve	
LA appendage: Check no clot that could be dislodged	
Presence of pericardial effusion pre-procedure	

Table 16.5 **Checklist in VSD**

Position, size (anatomical and physiological), and direction of shunt and margins
LV size and evidence of overload
PA pressure
Other congenital or acquired defects.
Distance from aortic valve—suitable for device closure?
Aneurysmal tissue associated with septal leaflet of tricuspid valve?

- The possible late complications of a small VSD are:
  - Increase in flow across the VSD because of increased LV pressures.
  - Jet lesion causing hypertrophy of the RV, leading to a double-chambered RV.
  - Progressive aortic regurgitation caused by prolapse of the right or non-coronary aortic cusp.
  - Discrete subaortic stenosis.
  - Endocarditis (see Chapter 13).

- **Localise the site of the defect** (Figure 16.2):
  - **Perimembranous** (80%). In a parasternal short-axis view, it is adjacent to the tricuspid valve. It could involve the RV inlet or outlet.
  - **Muscular** (15–20%). These may be multiple.
  - **Doubly committed subarterial or juxta arterial** (5%). This may be associated with prolapse of the right or non-coronary cusp of

175

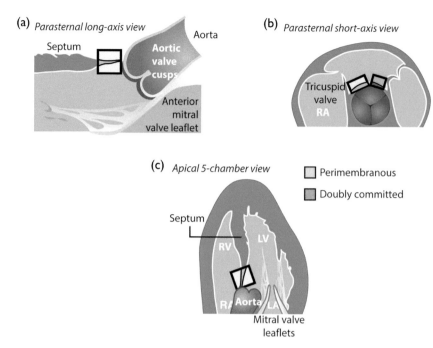

(a) *Parasternal long-axis view*

Septum

Aorta

Aortic valve cusps

Anterior mitral valve leaflet

(b) *Parasternal short-axis view*

Tricuspid valve

RA

(c) *Apical 5-chamber view*

☐ Perimembranous

☐ Doubly committed

Septum

RV

LV

RA

Aorta

LA

Mitral valve leaflets

Figure 16.2 **Position of ventricular septal defects.** (a) Parasternal short-axis at aortic level; (b) parasternal long-axis view; (c) apical 5-chamber.

the aortic valve. In a parasternal short-axis view, it is inferior to the pulmonary valve in a 12–3 o'clock position.

- **Atrioventricular septal defect** (Table 16.3).
- **Gerbode defect,** which is a shunt between the LVOT and right atrium. This is rare. The jet may be confused with TR.

- **Shunt direction?** In adult practice, this will usually be left to right, but if the pulmonary vascular resistance is high, flow may be right to left or bidirectional.
- **Estimate the size:**
  - A restrictive defect (LV pressure is significantly higher than RV pressure) is shown by a $V_{max} > 4.0$ m/s.
  - The shunt size can be estimated (Appendix, page 242) as a guide, but the LV size and activity are usually used as an indication for surgery in asymptomatic patients.
  - In the presence of pulmonary hypertension, a left-to-right shunt >1.5 and a PA systolic pressure (or pulmonary vascular resistance) <2/3 systemic levels suggest that surgery may still be considered[5].

- **Assess the LV.** LV volume load and systolic dilatation suggest a large shunt and are criteria for closure.
- **Assess the RV.** Hypertrophy of muscular bands may be associated with a perimembranous defect, causing a double-chambered RV.

- **Estimate pulmonary artery pressures** (Chapter 5).
  - Be careful to position the cursor away from VSD flow when recording TR V_{max}.
  - Usually, if the PA systolic pressure is >50% systemic pressure, it is advisable to measure PA pressures and resistance invasively before considering closure.

MISTAKES TO AVOID

- Forgetting to look for an ASD in a volume-loaded RV. Consider other imaging modalities (CT, CMR, TOE) to exclude sinus venosus defects and abnormal pulmonary venous drainage if no ASD was detected on TTE.
- Failing to recognise LV volume load with a VSD as an indication for surgery.
- Mistaking VSD flow on continuous wave Doppler for tricuspid regurgitation when calculating PA pressures.
- Missing a restrictive muscular defect towards the apex. This may be first detected using a continuous wave probe placed at the apex.
- Mistaking SVC flow for an ASD.

3. Persistent duct (PDA) (Table 16.6)

This is a channel between the proximal descending thoracic aorta and the origin of the left pulmonary branch. It is usually at or beyond the level of left subclavian artery.

- Look for reversed flow in the main pulmonary artery using parasternal short- and long-axis views and for the duct in the suprasternal view (Figure 16.3a).
- Estimate pulmonary artery pressure. When normal, flow is continuous throughout the cardiac cycle (Figure 16.3b). When raised, flow through the duct may diminish, cease, or reverse during systole.
- The shunt size can be estimated (Appendix, page 242) as a guide, but LV volume load suggests a large shunt.

Table 16.6 Checklist in persistent duct

Size and direction of flow
LV size and function (volume load in moderate or large persistent duct)
PA size (commonly dilated)
RV function (pressure load with Eisenmenger physiology) and pulmonary artery pressure
Other congenital or acquired defects?
Coarctation or tapering of the descending aorta?

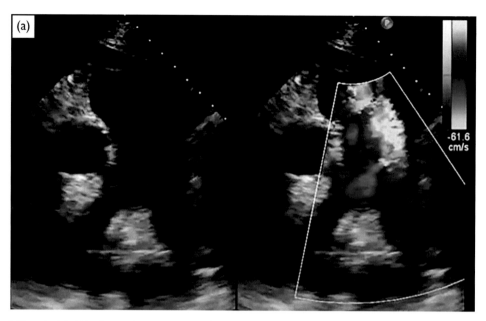

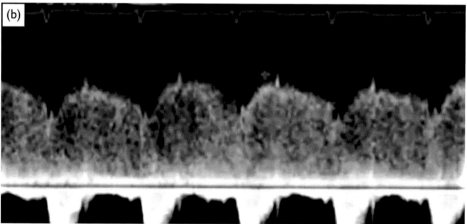

Figure 16.3 **Persistent ductus.** A large duct with normal pulmonary pressures imaged from a parasternal short-axis view with and without colour Doppler (a) and on continuous wave Doppler (b).

4.   **Coarctation** (Table 16.7)
   ● This is a narrowing of the aorta, usually just beyond the left subclavian artery at the site of the ductus arteriosus.
   ● Always check for coarctation in patients with:
       ● Bicuspid aortic valve
       ● Early-onset systemic hypertension
       ● Murmur
       ● Syndromes associated with coarctation (Turner, Williams, congenital rubella, neurofibromatosis)

- **Appearance**
  - Describe the site and appearance (membrane, tunnel, S-shape) using imaging and colour flow assessment.
  - Measure aortic dimensions above and below the coarctation.
  - Look for associated aortic root dilatation and bicuspid aortic valve.
  - Check for LV hypertrophy and assess LV systolic and diastolic function.

- **Continuous wave Doppler**
  - The most reliable feature on continuous wave recording is forward flow during diastole (Figure 16.4).

- Elevated flow velocities are usually seen in systole but may occasionally be absent or difficult to record if there is a severe or complete coarctation with extensive collaterals.

Table 16.7 **Checklist in coarctation**

Site and morphology (membrane, tunnel, S-shape).
Systolic and diastolic flow.
Presence of bicuspid valve?
Diameter of aorta at all levels, ascending and descending thoracic and abdominal.
LV adaptation, especially hypertrophy, systolic, and diastolic function.
Other congenital or acquired defects.

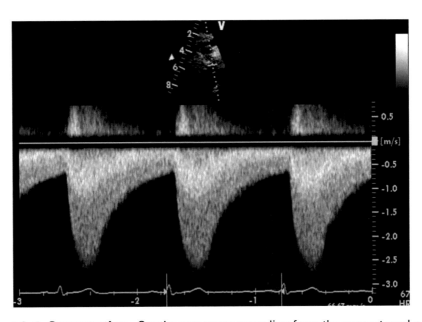

Figure 16.4 **Coarctation.** Continuous wave recording from the suprasternal notch.

- Intervention is not decided by the velocities or gradients across the coarctation but by the presence of systemic hypertension and:
  - A pressure difference >20 mmHg between upper and lower limbs, or
  - Narrowing ≥50% relative to aortic diameter at diaphragm level on CT or CMR.

5. **Ebstein's anomaly** (Table 16.8)
   - This is characterised by:
     - Apical displacement of the septal/posterior leaflets of the tricuspid valve towards the apex. The distance between the mitral annulus and the base of the displaced leaflet indexed to BSA (displacement index) must be >8 mm/m².
     - An elongated anterior leaflet meeting the septal leaflet.
     - Division of the RV into an atrialised portion and a residual functional RV.
     - Associated tricuspid regurgitation.
   - The diagnosis is often suspected from a combination of:
     - Right-sided dilatation in the parasternal views.
     - Tricuspid regurgitation originating more apically than normal on the apical 4-chamber view.
   - The haemodynamic effect of the anomaly is related to:
     - The size and function of the residual functional RV
     - The degree of tricuspid regurgitation.
     - The presence of other congenital defects, especially ASD, which occurs in about 1/3 of cases.
   - Surgery is indicated[1, 6] for:
     - Symptoms and more than moderate TR.
     - Progressive right-sided dilatation or reduction in RV function.

Table 16.8 Checklist in Ebstein's anomaly

Degree of apical displacement of the septal and posterior leaflets.
Degree of tethering of the anterior leaflet to the free wall, which affects the ability to repair the valve.
Grade of tricuspid regurgitation?
Size of the residual functional RV—if >1/3 total, makes repair more likely.
Function of the residual RV.
Are there associated congenital defects? 1/3 have ASD, 10% have left-sided abnormalities, for example, cor triatriatum, cleft mitral valve, parachute mitral valve, bicuspid aortic valve. Other defects include congenitally corrected transposition, and pulmonary outflow stenosis.

Table 16.9 **Echo features of congenitally corrected transposition**

Pulmonary artery and aorta in parallel on parasternal long-axis view
Both valves seen en face in a parasternal short-axis view
Ventricles reversed (morphological RV connected to the LA)
Dilated and hypertrophied morphological RV invariable
Left AV valve (tricuspid) regurgitation
Associated congenital defects (VSD, PS, malformations of the tricuspid valve, complete heart block)

- Isolated closure of ASD or PFO may be performed in systemic embolization, depending on RV function.

6. **Congenitally corrected transposition of the great arteries** (Table 16.9)
    - Just the ventricles are transposed:
        - The RA connects to a morphological LV and thence to the pulmonary artery.
        - The LA connects to a morphological RV and thence to the aorta.
    - This may present in adulthood. The key is that the systemic circulation is supplied by the morphological RV.
    - The morphological RV is always dilated and hypertrophied in response to the systemic pressure. Regurgitation of the left atrioventricular valve (tricuspid) may worsen ventricular function and require intervention.

Sequential Segmental Approach to Assessment of Congenital Heart Disease

- Congenital disease should be suspected if specific abnormalities are found (Table 16.10).
- You may have little or no background information (e.g. new diagnosis, emergency admission, details of corrective surgery not available).
- **Defining terms:**
    - **'Situs'** is the term used to define whether the heart and organs are correctly positioned. More specifically, it refers to the position of the atria relative to the great veins.
    - **'Atrioventricular valve'** refers to the tricuspid and mitral valves. The 'left atrioventricular valve' makes no assumptions that this is truly the mitral valve.
    - **'Semilunar valve'** refers to the pulmonary and aortic valves.

181

Table 16.10 **Findings suspicious of congenital disease**

Dilated or hypertrophied right ventricle
Pulmonary hypertension
Lack of AV valve offsetting in the 4-chamber view (endocardial cushion defect)
Abnormal AV valves offsetting (congenitally corrected transposition)
Pulmonary artery and aorta seen in parallel or pulmonary and aortic valves seen in the same parasternal short-axis view (congenitally corrected transposition)
Hyperdynamic LV without aortic or mitral regurgitation
Dilated coronary sinus (usually persistent left-sided SVC)

- **'Morphological left ventricle'** means the ventricle attached to the mitral valve.
- **'Systemic ventricle'** means the ventricle supplying the systemic circulation.
- **'Discordant'** means incorrect connections, for example, left atrium attached to morphological right ventricle or aorta leading from morphological right ventricle.

Perform a systematic study using a sequential segmental approach

1. **Define situs (are the atria correctly positioned?)**
   - The morphological left and right atria are distinguished by the relative position of the inferior vena cava (IVC) and abdominal aorta.
   - What is the position of the IVC and abdominal aorta in the subcostal short-axis view? The aorta normally lies posterior and to the left of the spine. The IVC lies anterior and to the right.
   - Follow the IVC (and SVC if visible) to the right atrium using subcostal views and check that this is on the correct side of the heart.
   - With situs anomalies or a right-sided aortic arch, the aorta may lie to the right of the spine and the IVC to the left.

2. **Is the heart correctly positioned?**
   - Position is defined by both:
     - Position of the heart: in the left chest, midline, right chest.
     - Position of the apex: apex to the left, apex to midline, apex to the right (apex to right: dextrocardia; heart in right chest but apex to left: dextroposition; apex in midline: mesocardiac).
   - Keep the probe marker in the normal orientation to allow for correct imaging interpretation on retrospective review.

3. **Are the atria attached to the correct ventricles?**
    - This is usually appreciated best from the apical 4-chamber view.
    - Atrioventricular connections can be[7]:
        - Concordant (e.g. right atrium to morphological RV).
        - Discordant (e.g. right atrium to morphological LV).
        - Absent (e.g. absent right atrioventricular connection).
        - Double-inlet connection (e.g. both atria open to a single dominant ventricle).
    - The morphological RV is recognised because:
        - Its atrioventricular valve inserts more towards the apex and has three leaflets (3D may be very helpful).
        - There is no continuity between the atrioventricular valve and the semilunar valve.

    Other helpful features are:
    - There are more trabeculations than in the morphological LV.
    - There is usually a moderator band (LV occasionally has a false tendon).
    - Chords attached to the septum.

4. **Are the ventricles attached to the correct great arteries?**
    - Ventriculoarterial connections can be[7]:
        - Concordant (e.g. morphological RV to pulmonary artery).
        - Discordant (e.g. morphological RV to aorta).
        - Absent (e.g. pulmonary atresia or aortic atresia).
        - Double outlet—both vessels arise from the same ventricle.
        - Common arterial trunk—a single vessel that gives rise to the coronary arteries and head and neck vessels but also the pulmonary arteries.
    - The pulmonary artery is recognised by its early bifurcation into left and right branches.
    - The aorta is recognised by giving off the coronary arteries and the head and neck branch arteries.

5. **Assess the size and systolic function of both ventricles** (Chapters 2 and 4)
    - It is usual for a morphological RV connected to the systemic circulation to be dilated and hypertrophied.

6. **Estimate pulmonary artery pressure** (Chapter 5)
    - Make sure to assess the atrioventricular valve jet from the ventricle connected to the pulmonary circulation.
    - If there is outflow obstruction from valve stenosis or a band, the calculated pressures will reflect ventricular and not pulmonary artery systolic pressure.

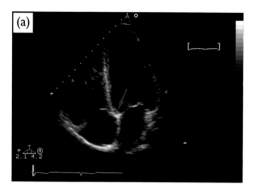
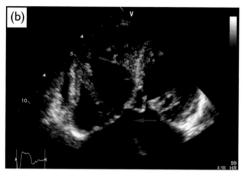

Figure 16.5 **Atrioventricular septal defect.** (a) A normal 4-chamber view showing that the tricuspid valve is offset or closer to the apex than the mitral valve. In (b), there is lack of offsetting, implying that there is a common AV valve. In addition, there is a large atrial septal defect (arrow).

7. **Are there any shunts at atrial or ventricular level?**
   - Measure size anatomically and estimate the shunt (page 242).

8. **Are the cardiac valves normal in appearance?**
   - Assess stenosis and regurgitation as for acquired valve disease.
   - If there is no offsetting of the atrioventricular valves, the diagnosis is likely to be atrioventricular septal defect (Figure 16.5). Check for a cleft in the left atrioventricular valve (anterior bridging leaflet).

9. **Is there aortic coarctation or a persistent duct** (pages 177 and 178)?

10. **Are the origins of the coronary arteries correctly positioned?**
    - In the parasternal short-axis view, the left coronary artery is usually seen at about 4 o'clock and the right at about 11 o'clock.

11. **Is the coronary sinus dilated?**
    - This is usually caused by a **persistent left-sided SVC** (image from the medial edge of the left supraclavicular fossa). A bubble study from the left arm will identify this.

Post-Procedure Studies

1. **Device closure for an ASD or patent foramen ovale** (Table 16.11)
   - Patients with residual shunts, raised PA pressure, or who have been repaired late should be followed at a specialist centre[1, 6].

2. **Closure of a VSD** (Table 16.12)
   - After device closure, follow-up every two to four years is recommended[1, 6].

3. **Closure of a persistent ductus** (Table 16.13)
   - Patients with no residual shunt, a normal LV, and normal PA pressure do not need follow-up beyond six months.
   - Patients with LV dysfunction or residual PA hypertension need follow-up at a specialist centre.

4. **Coarctation** (Table 16.14)
   - Long-term follow-up is recommended[1, 6].

5. **Tetralogy of Fallot** (Table 16.15)

Table 16.11 TTE Checklist after device closure of an ASD (Figure 16.6) or PFO

Device position
Is there any residual atrial shunt? Minor flow between the disks of the device is normal and will disappear with time.
Does the device obstruct the IVC or SVC or the pulmonary veins?
Is the device close to the mitral valve, and is there new or worse mitral regurgitation? Is there worse tricuspid regurgitation?
RV size and function (size may start to decrease soon after closure).
Pericardial effusion (as a sign of perforation during the procedure or early erosion).
PA pressure.
LV size and systolic function.

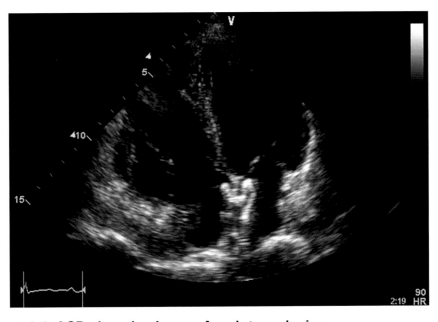

Figure 16.6 **ASD closed using an Amplatzer device.**

Table 16.12 **TTE after closure of a VSD**

Is there a residual shunt?
LV size and function.
Aortic regurgitation if closure of perimembranous VSD.
Pulmonary artery pressure.
Tricuspid regurgitation (septal leaflet most commonly damaged).

Table 16.13 **TTE after closure of a persistent duct**

Is there a residual shunt?
LV size and function.
Pulmonary artery pressure.
Associated lesions.

Table 16.14 **TTE after coarctation repair or stenting**

Is there a residual, new, or in-stent stenosis on imaging?
On continuous wave Doppler, an elevated systolic velocity is normal, but there should be no diastolic forward flow.
Assess the aorta beyond the repair, looking for aneurysmal dilatation.*
Assess the ascending aorta (which may be dilated) and aortic valve (may be bicuspid).
Assess LV size, function, and hypertrophy.

* Better performed with CMR.

Table 16.15 **TTE after repair of tetralogy of Fallot[7]**

RV size and function, including RV pressure.
Assess the RV outflow tract for muscular hypertrophy and/or aneurysm.
TR degree and mechanism: • Patch disrupting septal-anterior commissure   • Annular dilatation   • Organic abnormality of the valve   • Pacing electrode
RA size.
LV size (is there evidence of systolic dysfunction?).
Is the VSD patch competent, or is there a residual VSD?
Assess pulmonary valve for stenosis and regurgitation (especially if trans-annular PV patch was used).

Table 16.15 (Continued)

Assess branch pulmonary artery flow on colour and pulsed Doppler if possible. There may be a residual branch stenosis.
Size of aortic root and ascending aorta and 'sidedness' of aortic arch.
Degree of aortic regurgitation secondary to aortic dilatation.
Origin of coronary arteries.
Presence of systemic-to-pulmonary collateral vessels.
Presence of associated anomalies.

- The main diagnostic morphological features are:
  (a) Non-restrictive VSD with (b) overriding aorta
  (c) RV outflow obstruction (valvar or infundibular or both) with (d) RV hypertrophy
- The possible complications shown on TTE after repair are given in Table 16.15.

References

1. Baumgartner H, De Backer J, Babu-Narayan SV, et al. ESC 2020 Guidelines for the management of adult congenital heart disease. Europ Heart J 2021;42(6):563–645.
2. Verheugt CL, Uiterwaal CSPM, van der Velde ET, et al. Turning 18 with congenital heart disease: Prediction of infective endocarditis based on a very large population. Eur Heart J 2011;32(15):1926–34.
3. Valente AM, Cook S, Festa P, et al. Multimodality imaging guidelines for patients with repaired tetralogy of Fallot. J Am Soc Echo 2014;27(2):111–41.
4. Silvestry FE, Cohen MS, Laurie B. Armsby, et al. Guidelines for the echocardiographic assessment of atrial septal defect and patent foramen ovale: From the American Society of Echocardiography and Society for Cardiac Angiography and Interventions. J Am Soc Echo 2015;28(8):910–58.
5. Naqvi N, McCarthy KP & Ho SY. Anatomy of the atrial septum and interatrial communications. J Thoracic Dis 2018;10(Suppl 24):S2837–47.
6. Stout KK, Daniels CJ, Aboulhosn JA, Aboulhosn JA, et al. AHA/ACC 2018 Guideline for the management of adults with congenital heart disease: A report of the American College of Cardiology/American Heart Association Task Force on Clinical Practice Guidelines. J Am Coll Cardiol 2019;73(12):e81–192.
7. Bellsham-Revell H & Navroz Masani N. Educational series in congenital heart disease: The sequential segmental approach to assessment. Echo Research and Practice 2019;6(1):R1–8.

Pericardial Disease

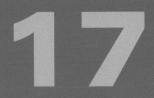

- Echocardiography is indicated for:
  - Pericardial effusion (Table 17.1).
  - Pericardial constriction.
  - Pericarditis (although this is diagnosed clinically, not on echocardiography).

- It may be used to guide percutaneous pericardiocentesis.

Pericardial Effusion

1. **Pericardial or pleural?**
   - The differentiation is usually obvious. The key is where the effusion ends in relation to the descending thoracic aorta (Table 17.2 and Figure 17.1).
   - The differentiation may be hard after cardiac surgery with a localised posterior effusion, particularly around the right atrium.
   - Pleural and pericardial effusions may coexist.

2. **Size, distribution and characteristics**
   - Pericardial fluid is always present, so a trivial effusion (Table 17.3) can be seen even in normal people, especially around the right atrium.
   - Size (Table 17.3) is graded semi-quantitatively, but whether there is evidence of tamponade (Table 17.4) is more important.
   - Small effusions may cause tamponade if acute (e.g. after instrumentation of the heart—pacing, ablation, coronary dissection) or if there is LV hypertrophy.
   - Is the effusion generalised or localised, for example, posterior, apical, or anterior?
   - Is there enough fluid in the subcostal view for safe pericardiocentesis (usually >20 mm)?
   - What is the consistency of the fluid?
     - Echolucent.
     - Localised strands which are common if the protein content is high, particularly in TB.

DOI: 10.1201/9781003242789-17

Table 17.1 **Cause of pericardial effusion**[1]

Common	
Infection	Viral (Coxsackievirus, echovirus, HIV), TB, Coxiella
Cancer	Angiosarcoma, metastases
Metabolic	Low albumin, hypothyroidism, renal failure
Reactive	Chest infections, especially pneumococcal
Systemic inflammatory diseases	SLE, rheumatoid arthritis, Sjögren's syndrome, systemic sclerosis
Heart failure	
Idiopathic	
Uncommon	
Post-radiation	
Post-pericardiotomy (Dressler) syndrome	Autoimmune pericarditis, typically two to six weeks after cardiac surgery, myocardial infarction, or trauma
Direct injury	Blunt or sharp chest injury, ablation
Drugs	Isoniazid, minoxidil, hydralazine, phenytoin
Aortic dissection	

Table 17.2 **Differential diagnosis of pericardial and pleural effusions**

Pericardial	Pleural
Ends anterior to the descending aorta	Ends posterior to the descending aorta
Almost never overlaps left atrium	May overlap left atrium
Fluid between heart and diaphragm on subcostal view	No fluid between heart and diaphragm on subcostal view
Tamponade may be present	No signs of tamponade
Rarely >40 mm in depth	May often be >40 mm in depth
If large, swinging of the heart	Heart not mobile

Table 17.3 **Grading pericardial effusions by size**

Trivial	Parietal and visceral pericardium only separated in systole
Small	<10 mm at end-diastole
Moderate	10–20 mm at end-diastole
Large	>20 mm at end-diastole

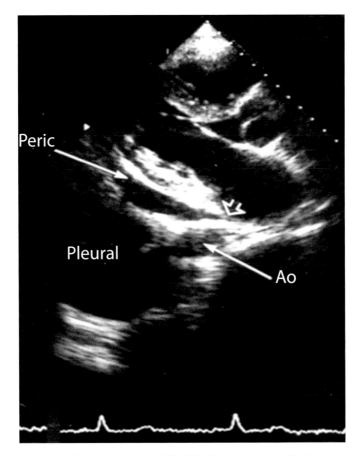

Figure 17.1 Pericardial vs pleural fluid. A pericardial effusion ends anterior to the descending thoracic aorta; a pleural effusion ends posterior to the aorta. A pleural effusion may extend over the left atrium, a pericardial effusion never does to any significant degree.

- Echodense—haematomas occur after cardiac surgery, chest trauma and aortic dissection.

- Are there reasons that drainage with a needle might not be feasible?
  - Too small.
  - Position (e.g. too posterior to reach percutaneously).
  - Loculated.
  - Echodense.

3. **Is tamponade present?**
    - Ultimately, this is a clinical diagnosis, but it is aided by the TTE (Table 17.4)[2].
    - In mechanical ventilation, the signs will be modified. Respiratory variation of echocardiographic measures is minimal or reversed with positive-pressure ventilation.

Table 17.4 **Echocardiographic evidence of tamponade**

Key signs
Fall in transmitral E wave (and aortic) velocity during inspiration >25% (Figure 17.2)[3]
Prolonged and widespread diastolic RV collapse
Dilated IVC (>20 mm) with inspiratory collapse <50% (Figure 17.3)
Other signs
Decrease in LV size on inspiration
Increase in trans-tricuspid velocities on inspiration >40%

Note: NB collapse of the right atrium and right ventricular outflow tract occurs before RV free wall collapse and is a nonspecific sign.

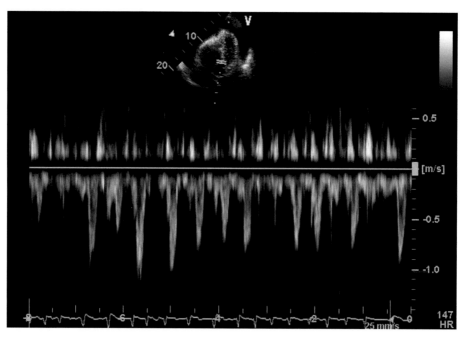

Figure 17.2 **Increased paradox.** This signal was recorded in a patient with tamponade. The subaortic peak velocity falls by >25% during inspiration.

- Tamponade may be caused by a regional pericardial effusion, particularly after cardiac surgery.
- The decision to drain an effusion may be based on:
  - Haemodynamic deterioration without another obvious cause
  - Presence of sufficient fluid on the TTE to drain safely

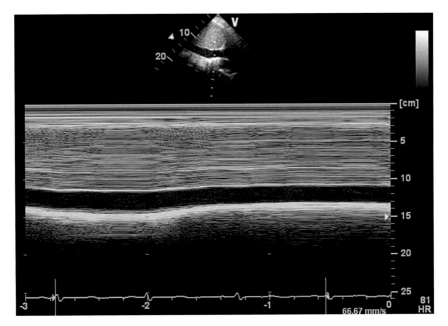

Figure 17.3 **Engorged inferior vena cava.** There is little change in diameter throughout the respiratory cycle or after a sniff.

- After cardiac surgery, there may be tamponade because of haematoma compressing the atria. TTE can be challenging, and diagnosis may require TOE.
- If there is tamponade despite a small effusion, especially if chronic (>3 months), consider effusive-constrictive pericarditis. This requires investigation as for pericardial constriction.

4.   **Differential diagnoses**
- The main differential diagnoses of pericardial fluid are:
  - Pleural fluid.
  - Fat, which most commonly occurs anteriorly or between the RV and diaphragm. It often has a brighter signal than the myocardium and fascial planes sliding across each other during the cardiac cycle. There may also be a little echolucent fluid.
  - Pericardial cyst (see page 210).
- Increased left-sided respiratory variation may also be caused by:
  - Asthma.
  - Right heart failure.
  - Circulatory underfilling.

193

5. **LV function**
- Is LV function poor?
  - Pericardial effusions can complicate myocarditis.
  - Rapid total pericardiocentesis may cause circulatory collapse.
- Wall motion abnormalities may complicate tamponade even with normal coronary anatomy.

6. **Pericardiocentesis**
TTE can help with:
- Checking if there is sufficient fluid for safe pericardiocentesis.
- Measuring the depth of the effusion below the skin.
- Confirming the needle tip is in the fluid (reinject a little fluid to create bubble contrast).
- Confirming resolution of effusion.

Pericardial Constriction

- This needs to be considered in patients with clinical evidence of heart failure but normal LV ejection fraction.
- Causes of pericardial constriction are tuberculosis, radiation, post-viral, rheumatoid arthritis, idiopathic, and rarely, after cardiac surgery.
- The key to the physiology is that the ventricles are normal but surrounded by a rigid 'box', causing:
  - Increased ventricular interdependence (i.e. as the RV gets bigger on inspiration, the LV must get smaller).
  - On inspiration, the fall in intrathoracic pressure is not transmitted inside the pericardium, so pulmonary venous flow and, therefore, left-sided velocities drop.
- Visual assessment in suspected pericardial constriction is given in Table 17.5 and Doppler assessment in Table 17.6.

Table 17.5 **Visual assessment in pericardial constriction**

Septal bounce (Figure 17.4). Often the first clue. Caused by an early diastolic pressure rise in the RV[4].
Inspiratory septal shift. The interventricular septum deviates towards the LV during inspiration.
Pericardial thickening. Not reliably detected or excluded on TTE, but extensive thickening may still alert to the diagnosis. Thickness is better measured on CT.
Atrial size. Mild or moderate biatrial enlargement.
IVC. Dilated with reduced contraction on inspiration.

Table 17.6 **Doppler assessment in pericardial constriction**

Key signs
LV filling pattern. Characteristically restrictive (E/A ratio >2 and E deceleration time <150 ms) (Figure 17.5a).
Respiratory variability (in spontaneous respiration). Record the transmitral E wave or the peak transaortic velocities. Subtract the lowest (inspiratory) from the highest (expiratory) velocity and express as a percentage of the highest velocity. This is characteristically increased by >25% (Figure 17.5a).
Tissue Doppler. Normal S′ and normal or raised E′ velocities are characteristic. The peak E′ velocity may be higher at the septal than the lateral annulus (which may become tethered to the pericardium).
Estimated PA pressure. This is moderately increased (usually to <50 mmHg).
Other signs
Hepatic vein flow. Flow reversal is maximal on the first beat after expiration.
Pulmonary vein flow. A systolic-to-diastolic (S/D) velocity ratio >0.65 on inspiration and a D velocity fall by >40% on inspiration are characteristic.

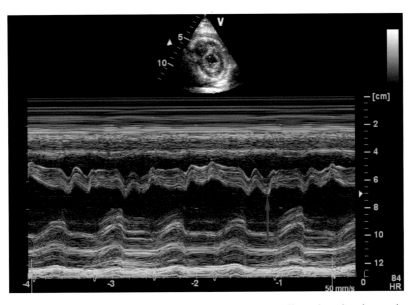

Figure 17.4 **Septal bounce.** This is an M-mode recording showing inward motion of the septum in systole but also diastole (the bounce).

And here's an electronic link to a loop on the website or use
http://goo.gl/Iw5YNB

And here's an electronic link to a loop on the website or use
http://goo.gl/Qo7Jlz

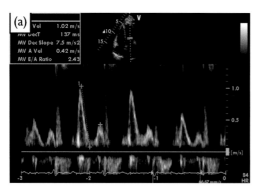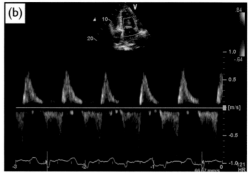

Figure 17.5 **Differentiating pericardial constriction and constrictive cardiomyopathy.** (a) This was recorded in a patient with pericardial constriction. The transmitral E deceleration time was 137 ms, and the peak E velocity fell by around 50% on inspiration. (b) This was recorded in a patient with amyloid secondary to multiple myeloma. The E wave varies little throughout the respiratory cycle.

1. **Pericardial constriction or restrictive cardiomyopathy?**
   - The distinction is important because the treatments are different. Constriction is potentially curable with surgery.
   - Many of the causes of pericardial constriction also affect the myocardium, so constriction and restrictive cardiomyopathy may coexist, and it is necessary to determine which is dominant.
   - The key is that the ventricles are normal in constrictive pericarditis but abnormal in restrictive cardiomyopathy (Table 17.7).

2. **Other imaging modalities:** [5–7]
   - **CMR or CT** are needed if a definitive diagnosis cannot be made on TTE. Where uncertainty remains, a left and right heart catheter study is indicated. Uncertainty is particularly likely if the RR interval is variable (e.g. AF or atrial ectopics).

Acute Pericarditis

- Acute pericarditis is a clinical diagnosis[8], but a basic TTE is usually recommended[7] to:
  - Detect pericardial effusion and tamponade.
  - Exclude regional or global LV dysfunction (myocarditis or acute coronary syndrome).
- Occasionally, the TTE may provide diagnostic clues, for example, valve involvement in SLE.

Table 17.7 **Differentiating pericardial constriction and restrictive cardiomyopathy**

Common to both		
Normal LV size and usually normal ejection fraction		
Restrictive transmitral physiology (E/A >2 and E dec <150 ms) (Figure 17.5)		
Dilated unreactive IVC (Figure 17.3)		
Points differentiating constriction and restrictive cardiomyopathy		
	Constriction	Restrictive cardiomyopathy
Myocardial appearance	Normal	LV ± RV hypertrophy or unusual echotexture
Pericardial thickness	Thickened pericardium or hyperechogenicity	Normal
Fall in transmitral E velocity or aortic velocity on inspiration (Figure 17.5)[3,5]	>25%	<15%
Tissue Doppler septal E'[5]	≥8 cm/s	<6 cm/s
LA and RA dilatation	Mild or moderate	Severe
Septal bounce (Figure 17.4)	Present	Absent
Septal shift toward LV in inspiration	Present	Absent
Hepatic flow reversal	Expiration	Inspiration
GLS	Normal	Reduced
PA systolic pressure	<50 mmHg	May be >50 mmHg

Table 17.8 **Other imaging modalities**

Cardiac magnetic resonance
Less accurate than CT for pericardial thickness but can identify pericardial inflammation
Better tissue characterisation than echocardiography for pericardial masses and for contents of the effusion (blood vs fluid)
CT
Measures pericardial thickness (abnormal if >4 mm), although a normal thickness does not exclude constriction
Detects calcification and masses
Evaluates the rest of the chest for evidence of malignancy and other lung pathology

197

MISTAKES TO AVOID

- Failing to image subcostally to check that there is sufficient depth of pericardial effusion to allow safe pericardiocentesis.
- Forgetting to check for a septal 'bounce', dilated IVC, and short transmitral E deceleration time in a patient with clinical heart failure but normal LV size and ejection fraction.
- Diagnosing epicardial fat as a pericardial effusion.

CHECKLIST REPORT IN PERICARDIAL DISEASE

1. Pericardial effusion.
   a. Size and site.
   b. Consistency.
   c. Is there fluid in the subcostal approach?
2. RV collapse.
3. LV size and function, including septal 'bounce', transmitral filling pattern, and respiratory variability.
4. Tissue Doppler at the septal mitral annulus.
5. PA pressure.
6. IVC size and response to inspiration.
7. Atrial size.

References

1. Imazio M & Adler Y. Management of pericardial effusion. Eur Heart J. 2013;34(16):1186–97.
2. Fowler N. Cardiac tamponade—A clinical or an echocardiographic diagnosis? Circulation 1993;87(5):1738–41.
3. Goldstein JA. Cardiac tamponade, constrictive pericarditis, and restrictive cardiomyopathy. Curr Probl Cardiol 2004;29(9):503–67.
4. Coylewright M, Welch TD & Nishimura RA. Mechanism of septal bounce in constrictive pericarditis: A simultaneous cardiac catheterisation and echocardiographic study. Heart 2013;99(18):1376.
5. Habib G, Bucciarelli-Ducci C, Caforio ALP, et al. Multimodality imaging in restrictive cardiomyopathies: An EACVI expert consensus document in collaboration with the 'Working Group on Myocardial and Pericardial Diseases' of the European Society

of Cardiology endorsed by the Indian Academy of Echocardiography. Eur Heart J CVI 2017;18(10):1090–1.

6. Klein AL, Abbara S, Agler DA, et al. American Society of Echocardiography Clinical Recommendations for Multimodality Cardiovascular Imaging of Patients with Pericardial Disease: Endorsed by the Society for Cardiovascular Magnetic Resonance and Society of Cardiovascular Computed Tomography. J Am Soc Echocardiogr 2013;26(9):965–1012.

7. Cosyns B, Plein S, Nihoyanopoulos P, et al. European Association of Cardiovascular Imaging (EACVI) position paper: Multimodality imaging in pericardial disease. Eur Heart J Cardiovasc Imaging 2015;16(1):12–31.

8. Chiabrando JG, Bonaventura A, Vecchié A, et al. Management of acute and recurrent pericarditis: JACC State-of-the-art review. J Am Coll Cardiol 2020;75(1):76–92.

Masses

18

- The aim is to differentiate between thrombus, vegetation, tumour, and normal findings.
- Secondary tumours are at least 20 times more common than primary tumours of the heart[1, 2].
- The most common benign primary tumours are atrial myxoma (70%), papillary fibroelastoma (10%), fibroma, and mainly in infants and children, rhabdomyoma[1, 2].
- The most common primary malignancies are the sarcomas, especially angiosarcomas, which usually arise in the RA. Lymphomas are less common.

Describe the Basic Characteristics of the Mass (Table 18.1)

The site of attachment and shape may be more easily appreciated using 3D echo.

Table 18.1 **Characteristics of the mass**

Site of attachment
Size, shape
Density (low intensity, dense, mixed)
Mobility (fixed, mobile, free)
Evidence of invasiveness, including pericardial involvement

Mass Attached to a Valve

- This can be solid or thin (Table 18.2).
- It is not possible to differentiate reliably a vegetation from a myxomatous mitral valve with ruptured chords. The TTE has to be interpreted within the clinical context.
- Echogenicity related to a valve annulus:
  - Mitral annular calcification: occasionally large and mistaken for an abnormal mass.
  - Fat in the tricuspid annulus: this is normal.

201

DOI: 10.1201/9781003242789-18

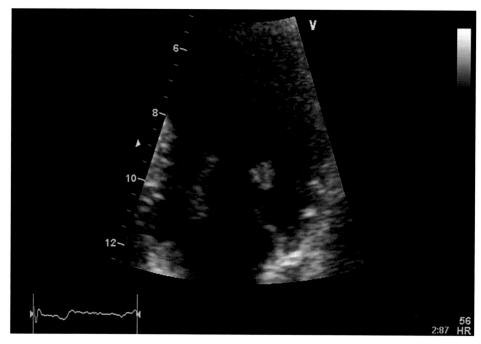

Figure 18.1 **Fibroelastoma.** An apical 4-chamber view showing a small pedunculated mass of mixed echogenicity is attached to the posterior leaflet of the mitral valve.

And here's an electronic link to a loop on the website or use http://goo.gl/X6G9Lf

Left or Right Atrial Mass

- Many apparent masses are normal (Table 18.3). Pathological masses are listed in Table 18.4.
- **For an RA mass:**
  - An associated pericardial effusion suggests an angiosarcoma (Figure 18.2).
  - Check the IVC for tumour extension from a primary tumour in the kidneys, liver, uterus, or ovaries.
  - Thrombus from a DVT may also appear in the IVC. Typically, a tumour will cause IVC dilatation (Figure 18.3), while a thrombus will not.
- **For an LA mass:**
  - If immobile and attached to the wall, check the pulmonary veins and look for a tumour mass outside the heart.
  - Thrombus is unlikely without a substrate (dilated LA, mitral stenosis, atrial fibrillation).

Table 18.2 **Masses attached to valves**

Native valves	
Solid mass	
Vegetation	Infective: Occurs on any valve, usually moving independently of the valve and associated with valve destruction.
	Libman–Sacks in SLE or isolated antiphospholipid syndrome: Usually broad-based, <10 mm in diameter, attached to aortic or mitral valves and associated with generalised thickening. May be calcified when chronic.
	Malignant: Indistinguishable from infective vegetations, but valve destruction less common.
	Other: rheumatoid arthritis.
Fibroelastoma	Small (usually <10 mm), with a short stalk, rounded with fronds, often with mixed echogenicity. Attached to the aortic > mitral valve > pulmonary or tricuspid valves (Figure 18.1).
Myxomatous tissue	Usually generalised mild 'fleshiness' associated with prolapse but may be florid in Barlow's syndrome. Mainly affects the mitral valve, less commonly the tricuspid valve.
Calcific deposit	The edges of atherosclerotic degeneration may be 'furry'. Atheroma may occasionally be pedunculated
Thin mass	
Single ruptured chord	This produces a whip-like appearance most often seen in the LA and moving between LA and LV.
Fibrin strand	Also called Lambl's excrescences. These are attached to the closure line of the aortic valve.
Replacement valves	
Solid mass	
Thrombus	This is more common in mechanical valves and requires TOE for full delineation.
Vegetation	These may be attached to the cusps of a biological valve or the sewing ring of any design.
Other	In old valves, disruption of the fabric covering the sewing ring or endothelial tags can rarely cause noninfected masses attached to the sewing ring.
Thin mass	
Stitch	These may be obvious around the sewing ring on TOE, occasionally on TTE.
Fibrin strand	These are seen mainly in mechanical valves and consist of 10–20 mm strands attached to the leaflets and wriggling.

Table 18.3 **Non-pathological atrial 'masses'**

Eustachian valve	Attached at the opening of the IVC, this can be fixed or mobile, thin or thick, and up to 20 mm in length.
Chiari membrane or network	Attached between the Eustachian valve and the atrial septum. Thin and may move gently.
Crista terminalis	May look like a mass if the RA is scanned obliquely in the 4-chamber view.
Atrial septal aneurysm	The apex may initially be seen as an apparent mass in the LA in parasternal long-axis views, although the diagnosis is obvious in other views.
Atrial septal fat	This is deposited in a dumb-bell shape at either end of the septum and sparing the centre.
Pacemaker electrode	Sections of the electrode will lie outside the plane of the ultrasound so requires multiple views.
Long central line	Usually, the 'railway track' appearance of the cannula is obvious.

Table 18.4 **Pathological atrial masses**

Location	Characteristics
Intracavitary	Fixed band across LA in cor triatriatum.
	Mobile mass in RA: Thrombus or tumour entering via IVC or thrombus wedged in PFO.
	Free-floating ball thrombus in the LA (associated AF and mitral stenosis).
Septum	Myxoma: Attached at the centre on the left much more commonly than the right. Mixed echogenicity. When large, may prolapse through the mitral valve in diastole or prevent full closure in systole.
	Thrombus: A vein cast may become embedded in a PFO and may be seen in both RA and LA.
LA appendage	95% of LA thrombus starts here and may be seen in a 2-chamber apical view on TTE but usually requires TOE for detection.
LA or RA Wall	Thrombus: Commonly around the LA appendage or at the most basal part of the LA between the pulmonary veins or of the RA between the IVC and SVC in a 4-chamber view.
	Tumour: A sessile immobile mass attached to the free wall of the RA is often an angiosarcoma (Figure 18.2).

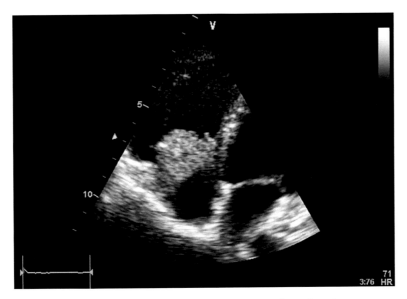

Figure 18.2 **Angiosarcoma.** An off-axis 4-chamber view showing a mass attached to the free wall of the right atrium. This is the most common malignant cardiac tumour and may often be associated with a pericardial effusion.

 And here's an electronic link to a loop on the website or use
http://goo.gl/5YB8z6

Left or Right Ventricular Mass

- See Table 18.5.
- An associated pericardial effusion suggests that the mass is malignant.
- LV thrombus is rare without an underlying structural abnormality (e.g. dilated LV, hypertrabeculation, regional wall motion abnormality) but may occur in a normal LV if there is thrombophilia (e.g. primary biliary cirrhosis, Behçet's disease).
- RV thrombus may complicate deep vein thrombosis or occur as a complication of an RV cardiomyopathy.
- If the presence of a thrombus is uncertain, use different views and consider transpulmonary contrast.
- Could the mass be normal (Table 18.7)?

Table 18.5 **Causes of LV or RV masses**

Intracavitary	
Thrombus	Table 18.6
Endomyocardial fibrosis	Causes thrombus at the apex of RV and LV (Figure 7.2, page 73) which may extend to the base of the heart and involve the AV valves.
Hypertrabeculation	Occurs predominantly in non-compaction (Figure 7.3, page 74).
Benign tumours	Fibroelastomas and myxomas may occasionally occur in the LV or RV.
Solely or predominantly intramyocardial	
Metastasis	Occur anywhere in LV or RV wall and may then extend inwards or outwards. Most commonly from breast, lung, stomach, and colonic carcinoma. Also occur with melanoma, germ cell carcinoma, thymoma.
Primary malignancy	Lymphomas or sarcomas extend outwards and may be associated with a pericardial effusion.
Fibroma	Usually in the septum or LV free wall. May be up to 100 mm in diameter. Characteristic central calcification (Figure 18.4).
Rhabdomyoma	Multiple bright intramural masses often extending into the cavity. Usually resolve in childhood.
Systemic disease	Myocardial nodules can occur in sarcoid, TB, or rheumatoid arthritis.
Hydatid disease[3]	Cystic, semisolid, or solid. Single or multiple. Also seen in the pericardium.

Table 18.6 **Features of thrombus**

Underlying wall motion abnormality
Cleavage plane between thrombus and LV wall
Higher density than myocardium
Present in more than one view
Causes a void on colour mapping or contrast echocardiography

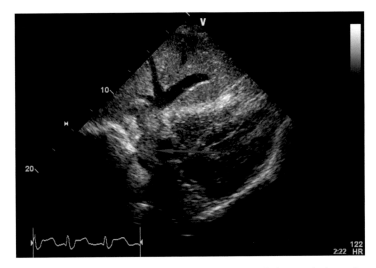

Figure 18.3 **Tumour in the inferior vena cava.** Subcostal view showing a large tumour mass stretching the inferior vena cava and entering the right atrium.

And here's an electronic link to a loop on the website or use
http://goo.gl/lyfK0e

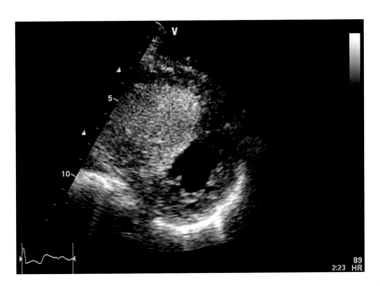

Figure 18.4 **Fibroma.** Parasternal short-axis view showing a large intramyocardial mass which is distinct from the surrounding myocardium.

And here's an electronic link to a loop on the website or use
http://goo.gl/iW0932

Table 18.7 **Normal LV or RV 'masses'**

Trabeculation	Trabeculation is a feature of the RV, and minor trabeculation is also common in the LV and increases with athletic training, especially in Afro-Caribbean people.
Prominent moderator band	Normal feature of the RV.
LV false tendon	Runs parallel with the septal endocardium.
Prominent papillary muscle	An occasional cause of confusion resolved by following back the apparent mass to show continuity with LV wall and chords.
Aberrant papillary muscles	Ectopic extra papillary tissue is sometimes seen (e.g. in the LVOT).
Near-field effects at the apex	Not seen in every view. Resolves with changes in focus and gain. Occasionally need contrast to resolve.

Pericardial Mass

- Apparent pericardial masses associated with a pericardial effusion are often proteinaceous deposits over the pericardium rather than true masses. These are especially common with TB or bleeding (e.g. pericarditis on heparin).
- True masses caused by tumour deposits within the pericardium may cause:
  - Generalised thickening of the pericardium (metastatic disease).
  - Localised tumour mass (primary tumours or less commonly, solitary metastasis).
  - An associated pericardial effusion.

- Look for:
  - Invasion of the underlying myocardium.
  - Constrictive physiology.

Extrinsic Mass

Table 18.8 **Masses outside the heart**

Diagnosis	Note
Abnormal findings	
Mediastinal tumour	Commonly lymphoma (Figure 18.5).
Lymph node	Most common adjacent to the pulmonary artery.
Haematoma	Tissue characterisation on CT and CMR.
Pericardial cyst	Table 18.9.

Table 18.8 (Continued)

Diagnosis	Note
Pericardial hydatid[3]	Rare (far more common in LV or RV). May be single or multiloculated or solid. Suspect according to background disease prevalence. Needs CT or MRI.
Pseudoaneurysm	Not usually a diagnostic problem with an associated myocardial infarct.
Subdiaphragmatic masses	Polycystic disease affecting the kidney or individual cysts of the liver should be reported as incidental findings.
Normal findings confused with masses	
Descending thoracic aorta	Continuity of structure in all views. Contains blood flow.
Hiatus hernia	Mixed echogenicity. Can be enhanced by the patient drinking a fizzy drink.
Back bone	May be especially prominent in a patient with pectus excavatum.
Pericardial fat	Seen most commonly anteriorly in a parasternal long-axis view and between the diaphragm and RV subcostally.

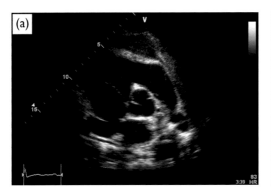
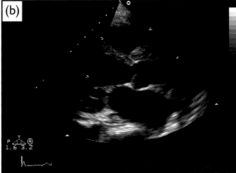

Figure 18.5 **Lymphoma.** This is a parasternal short-axis view showing a mediastinal mass (a) that extends down the anterior aorta in a long-axis view (b).

And here's an electronic link to a loop on the website or use
http://goo.gl/vt0xV4

Table 18.9 **Differentiating a pericardial cyst from a localised effusion**

	Pericardial cyst	Localised effusion
Circumstance	Incidental finding	May be after cardiac surgery or pericarditis
Position	Commonly right (50–70%) > left costophrenic angle (30–40%)	Cardiac border
Shape	Well-circumscribed and ovoid	More diffuse and crescentic
Effect of respiration	Shape may change	Fixed

Mass in the Great Vessels

1. **Haemodynamic effect**
   - Assess the presence and degree of valve regurgitation or obstruction to inflow, depending on the site of the mass.

2. **Other features**

Diagnosis of the mass may also be aided by:
   - Presence of a pericardial effusion, suggesting malignancy.
   - Substrate for thrombus formation: atrial fibrillation; enlarged LA; mitral stenosis; dilated hypokinetic LV; regional wall motion abnormality.

Table 18.10 **Masses in the great arteries**

Pulmonary artery	
Thrombus	Associated with deep vein thrombosis and pulmonary embolism
Sarcoma	Rare
Myxoma	Very rare
Aortic	
Dissection	Serpiginous motion of a flap in a dilated aorta is usually obvious, but a localised dissection after instrumentation may produce a small focal thickening.
Pedunculated atheroma	Most commonly seen on TOE.
Fungal aortitis	Rare complication of cardiac surgery. Classical appearance of large vegetation attached to the aortic wall at the site of the aortotomy.

- Medical history, for example, cancer, pulmonary embolism, evidence of infective endocarditis.

3. Other imaging modalities (Table 18.11)

If characterisation is difficult, consider other techniques.

Table 18.11 **Other techniques for characterising cardiac masses[4]**

Technique	Value
Contrast Echo	Confirms presence and site Demonstrates vascularity
TOE	Improves characterisation of all atrial masses
CMR	Improves tissue characterisation May differentiate thrombus from myxoma Can confirm presence of cardiac lipomas Perfusion (vascularity of masses)
PET	Demonstrates metabolic activity in malignancy and involvement of other organs
CT	Mediastinal extent and involvement of other organs; demonstrates local invasion

 # MISTAKES TO AVOID

- Overdiagnosing normal variants as abnormal.
- Failing to check the IVC if there is a right atrial mass.
- Ignoring the clinical background when suggesting the nature of a mass, for example, the presence of atrial fibrillation, especially with atrial or LV dilatation, makes thrombus more likely than tumour.

CHECKLIST REPORT FOR A MASS

1. Location and site of attachment.
2. Size, density, and mobility.
3. Involvement of adjacent veins and evidence of invasion.
4. Haemodynamic effect.
5. Is there a pericardial effusion?
6. Is there a substrate for thrombus?

References

1. Lam KY, Dickens P & Chan AC. Tumors of the heart. A 20-year experience with a review of 12,485 consecutive autopsies. Arch Pathol Lab Med 1993;117(10):1027–31.
2. Butany J, Nair V, Naseemuddin A, et al. Cardiac tumours: Diagnosis and management. Lancet Oncol 2005;6(4):219–28.
3. Dursun M, Terzibasioglu E, Yilmaz R, et al. Pictorial essay. Cardiac hydatid disease: CT and MRI findings. Am J Roentgenology 2008;190:226–32.
4. Klein AL, Abbara S, Agler DA, et al. American Society of Echocardiography Clinical Recommendations for Multimodality Cardiovascular Imaging of Patients with Pericardial Disease: Endorsed by the Society for Cardiovascular Magnetic Resonance and Society of Cardiovascular Computed Tomography. J Am Soc Echocardiogr 2013;26(9):965–1012.

Echocardiography in Acute and Critical Care Medicine

19

The Critically Ill Patient

- A cardiac ultrasound scan is used by the resuscitation team to detect:
  - Reversible causes (e.g. tamponade, pulmonary embolism, severe hypovolaemia).
  - The presence of myocardial contraction during cardiac arrest (10–35% of patients in asystole), which is associated with higher survival rates.
  - Pathology suggesting that prolonged resuscitation is likely to be futile (e.g. cardiac rupture).
- If time allows in critically ill medical patients, a basic echocardiogram (which includes colour) extends the diagnostic range to include shunts and valve disease (Table 19.1).
- All basic scans can be extended according to the clinical and echocardiographic findings, for example, the addition of TR V_{max} further improves the detection of pulmonary embolism (Table 19.2).

The Acutely Ill Patient

- **Haemodynamic instability after myocardial infarction** (Table 19.1)
- **Possible pulmonary embolism** (Table 19.2)
- **Unexplained severe hypotension** (Table 19.3)
- **Pulmonary oedema** (Table 19.4)
- **Chest pain where aortic dissection is suspected** (Table 19.5)
- **Trauma** (Table 19.6)
- **Acute exacerbation of COPD**. While not usually a critical emergency, 20% may have LV failure[1] so that early TTE may lead to an important change in management.

DOI: 10.1201/9781003242789-19

Table 19.1 Checklist for basic echocardiography in critically ill patients

Pericardial tamponade
Acute complications of infarction ● Papillary muscle rupture ● Ventricular septal rupture* ● Free wall rupture*
LV hypertrophy suggesting HCM
RV dilatation and dysfunction (e.g. secondary to pulmonary embolism; see Table 19.2)
Critical valve disease, especially aortic stenosis
Obstructed prosthetic valve*
Aortic dissection rupturing into pleural space or abdominal cavity*
Gross hypovolaemia

* Likely to require a more detailed echocardiogram.

Table 19.2 Echocardiographic signs of pulmonary embolism with haemodynamic instability[2-4]

RV dilatation and free wall hypokinesis often with preserved contraction at the apex (McConnell's sign). Basal RV/LV ratio >1.0 in apical 4-chamber view.
D-shaped LV in parasternal short-axis view.
TR V_{max} usually <4.0 m/s*.
IVC dilated and unreactive.
Diminished RV longitudinal function: TAPSE <17 mm.
Pulmonary acceleration time <80 ms*.
Right heart thrombus.

* Requires a more detailed echocardiogram.

Table 19.3 Checklist in hypotension

Signs of underfilling
IVC <10 mm in diameter collapsing completely on inspiration
Small and active RV and LV ('kissing papillary muscles') on parasternal short-axis view
Low E and A waves on transmitral pulsed Doppler*
Respiratory variability in $VTI_{subaortic}$ > 20% (in the absence of other pathology, particularly pericardial effusion, RV dilatation, or asthma)*
Cardiogenic causes
LV global or regional systolic dysfunction*
Dynamic LVOT obstruction*
RV systolic dysfunction (see also Table 19.2)
Pericardial tamponade
Severe valve lesions*
IVC diameter >21 mm with <50% contraction on sniff

Table 19.3 (Continued)

Sepsis[5]
LV typically normal in size or mildly dilated with global hypokinesis, but all forms of impairment can occur Fluid-loading and inotropes may lead to hyperkinesis
RV mildly dilated and hypokinetic (in the presence of ARDS)

Hypotension after cardiac surgery
HCM-like physiology following: • Aortic valve replacement for aortic stenosis with small LV cavity, systolic anterior mitral valve motion, and LVOT acceleration • Systolic anterior mitral motion after mitral valve repair
Prosthetic valve regurgitation or obstruction (TOE)
Native valve dysfunction
Localised haematoma over atria (TOE) or small effusion elsewhere, causing acute tamponade
RV stunning post-bypass and/or ischaemia

* Likely to require a more detailed echocardiogram.

Table 19.4 **Pulmonary oedema**

Impaired LV systolic or diastolic function
Complications of a myocardial infarction: • Papillary muscle rupture • Ventricular septal rupture* • Contained free wall rupture
Severe native valve disease
Severe dysfunction of a prosthetic heart valve* (may need TOE)

* Likely to require a more detailed echocardiogram.

Table 19.5 **Chest pain**

Signs suggestive of or compatible with dissection:* • Dissection flap • Dilated ascending aorta • Severe aortic regurgitation • Pericardial fluid
Wall motion abnormalities suggesting acute coronary syndrome
Signs of pulmonary embolism (Table 19.2)

* If TTE normal but a high suspicion for dissection remains, consider TOE or CT.

Table 19.6 **Checklist for echocardiography after blunt or penetrating trauma**

Blunt
Pericardial effusion
Contusion: • RV dilatation and hypokinesis   • Localised LV thickening and wall motion abnormality, especially antero-apically
Ventricular septal rupture
Regional wall motion abnormality (from coronary artery dissection)
Deceleration
Valve rupture causing acute mitral or tricuspid regurgitation, occasionally aortic regurgitation
Aortic dilatation and dissection flap or intramural haematoma (CT or TOE)
Aortic transection (TOE)
Penetrating
RV wall hypokinesis
Ventricular septal defect
Pericardial effusion or haematoma (which may be localised)
Pleural fluid
Mitral regurgitation from valve laceration or damage to papillary muscle or chords
Aortic regurgitation from laceration of aortic valve
Hyperdynamic LV (from offloading)

Further Indications for Echocardiography on Critical Care Units

● The haemodynamic assessment of the heart is altered by mechanical ventilation (Table 19.7), so the diagnosis of tamponade is based more on clinical features than in a spontaneously breathing patient.

- In the presence of a pericardial effusion, a fall in blood pressure or cardiac output and/or the development of acute renal failure with no other reasonable cause should prompt consideration of drainage.

The following situations require focused TTE, sometimes with additional TOE:

- Hypotension after cardiac surgery (Table 19.3).
- Estimation of filling pressures, low in Table 19.3 and high in Table 19.8.
- Assessment of likely cardiac output response to increased filling.
- The response of the $VTI_{subaortic}$ to passive leg raising aids the decision for fluid resuscitation. A rise by $\geq 15\%$ suggests that cardiac output will rise after fluid administration[6]. The role of measuring variation in IVC diameter with respiration is less clear.

Table 19.7 Effects of mechanical ventilation[7]

The timing of paradox is reversed: a fall in left-sided cardiac output during expiration and a decrease in right-sided venous return during inspiration.
Respiratory variation may be greater than normal, depending on the inspiratory pressure, but if >25%: • Check ventilation settings. • Exclude a pericardial effusion. • Check LV and RV size and function. • Check for hypovolaemia.
High positive end-expiratory pressure (PEEP) reduces venous return and afterload to cause: • Reduced stroke volume. • Reduced E'. • Lengthening of E deceleration time. • RV dilatation and dysfunction if PEEP very high (>15 mmHg).

Table 19.8 Signs of high filling pressures

High RA pressure
IVC >21 mm in diameter and unresponsive or unreactive SVC on TOE
Dilated right atrium
Atrial septum bulges to the left throughout the cardiac cycle
High LA pressure
E/E' ratio >14
E dec time <150 ms
Atrial septum bulges to the right throughout the cardiac cycle
Dilated left atrium if filling pressure chronically high

Table 19.9 **Other common indications for echocardiography on critical care units**

Indication	Checklist*
Inability to wean from ventilator	LV systolic and diastolic dysfunction? A high LVEDP is the most common cause. RV size and dysfunction? Severe valve disease? Pericardial effusion?
Unexplained hypoxaemia	Evidence of pulmonary embolism (Table 19.2). Shunt: This requires a bubble study if an ASD is not obvious (pages 56, 57).
ARDS not responding to first-line measures	RV size and function. PA pressures.
Pre- and peri-administration of nitric oxide	RV function and PA pressures.
Pre- and post-inotrope	LV and RV function.
Possible endocarditis	Chapter 13.
Embolic event	Table 20.3.

* A full study looking for abnormalities in all parts of the heart is needed.

- Other common indications for critical care echocardiography are given in Table 19.8.
- The Appendix gives guides to the echocardiographic assessment on ECMO (Table s A.1–A.3), LV assist devices (Table A.4), and intra-aortic balloon pumps (Table A.5).

Echocardiography in COVID-19

- Cardiac involvement confers a high risk of mortality.
- The role of TTE is to:
  - Identify acute cardiac injury or hitherto-unknown but pre-existing cardiac dysfunction (Table 19.10).
  - Aid triage of patients.

- A focused TTE should suffice acutely (Chapter 1).
- Consult local and societal guidance for advice on protection of patient and sonographer and decontamination of ultrasound equipment.

Table 19.10 **Indications for echocardiography in COVID-19** (Figure 19.1)

Acute
Critically unwell (hypotension, pulmonary oedema, high oxygen requirements)
Evidence of cardiac involvement (elevated biomarkers, e.g. troponin, D-dimer, ferritin, BNP; ECG changes; cardiac symptoms)
Known cardiac disease
Follow-up: Inpatient
Monitor RV and LV function and pulmonary pressure if: • The baseline study is abnormal • When the patient is either not improving or deteriorating • When moving to rescue strategies (e.g. airway pressure release ventilation)
Follow-up: Outpatient
• Document resolution of acute abnormalities • New heart failure suspected

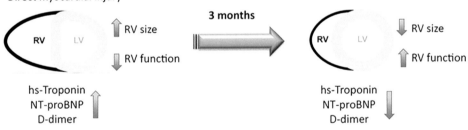

Acute COVID-19 disease
Hypoxic pulmonary vasoconstriction
Ventilator induced lung injury
Pulmonary thromboembolic disease
Direct myocardial injury

Recovery from COVID-19
Normalization of RV size and function

3 months

RV size
RV function
hs-Troponin
NT-proBNP
D-dimer

Figure 19.1 **Changes in COVID-19.** Right ventricular dilatation ± systolic dysfunction is the most common cardiac finding during acute, severe COVID-19 and may reverse with recovery. (Reproduced with permission from [9].)

CHECKLIST FOR REPORT IN COVID-19

1. LV dimensions, volume, and systolic function.
2. RV—dilatation and/or dysfunction and evidence of pulmonary hypertension.
3. Subclinical RV and/or LV dysfunction (e.g. longitudinal strain for outpatient cases with continuing exercise limitation).
4. Presence of incidental abnormalities (e.g. valve disease).
5. Pericardial and pleural effusions.

References

1. Rutten FH, Cramer MJM, Grobbee DE, et al. Unrecognized heart failure in elderly patients with stable chronic obstructive pulmonary disease. Eur Heart J. 2005;26(18):1887–94.
2. Kasper W, Geibel A, Tiede N, et al. Distinguishing between acute and subacute massive pulmonary embolism by conventional and Doppler echocardiography. Br Heart J 1993;70(4):352–6.
3. Kjaergaard J, Schaadt BK, Lund JO, et al. Quantitative measures of right ventricular dysfunction by echocardiography in the diagnosis of acute nonmassive pulmonary embolism. J Am Soc Echocardiogr 2006;19(10):1264–71.
4. McConnell M V, Solomon SD, Rayan ME, et al. Regional right ventricular dysfunction detected by echocardiography in acute pulmonary embolism. Am J Cardiol 1996;78(4):469–73.
5. Etchecopar-Chevreuil C, François B, Clavel M, et al. Cardiac morphological and functional changes during early septic shock: A transesophageal echocardiographic study. Intensive Care Med 2008;34(2):250–6.
6. Blanco P. Rationale for using the velocity-time integral and the minute distance for assessing the stroke volume and cardiac output in point-of-care settings. Ultrasound J 2020;12:21. doi.org/10.1186/s13089–020–00170-x.
7. Luecke T & Pelosi P. Clinical review: Positive end-expiratory pressure and cardiac output. Crit Care 2005;9(6):607–21.
8. Hothi SS, Jiang J, Steeds RP, et al. Utility of non-invasive cardiac imaging assessment in coronavirus disease 2019. Front Cardiovasc Med 2021;8:1–16.
9. Moody WE, Liu B, Mahmoud-Elsayed HM, et al. Persisting adverse ventricular remodeling in COVID-19 survivors: A longitudinal echocardiographic study. J Am Soc Echocardiogr 2021;34(5):562–6.

General Clinical Requests

These tables give guidance on what to assess in various common indications for echocardiography:

- Murmur (Table 20.1)
- Suspected heart failure (Table 20.2)
- Stroke, TIA, and peripheral embolism (Table 20.3)
- Hypertension (Table 20.4)
- Cardiac arrhythmia (Table 20.5)
- Cocaine (Table 20.6)
- HIV (Table 20.7)
- Neuromuscular diseases (Table 20.8)
- Inflammatory diseases (Table 20.9)
- Hypereosinophilia (Table 20.10)
- Drugs causing valvopathy: ergot alkaloids (cabergoline, pergolide), ergot dopamine agonists (pergolide and cabergoline), appetite suppressants (fenfluramine and dexfenfluramine), and the weight loss agent benfluorex (Table 20.11)
- Radiation (Table 20.12), mainly after treatment for non-Hodgkin's lymphoma or left-sided breast cancer more than 20 years ago

Table 20.1 **Checklist in murmur**

Valve thickening or regurgitation.
Subaortic septal bulge.
ASD: Clue is dilated active RV.
VSD: parasternal long- and short-axis views with colour box on the membranous septum detects most. Colour box over the septum in parasternal long- and short-axis and apical 4-chamber views. Apical septal defects may be missed (put CW probe over the site of the maximum murmur).
Aortic coarctation (suprasternal view).
Pulmonary valve/artery and branch stenosis (steerable continuous wave in pulmonary artery).
PDA (parasternal short and suprasternal views).

DOI: 10.1201/9781003242789-20

Table 20.2 **Checklist in suspected heart failure**

LV cavity size and wall thickness and systolic and diastolic function
RV size and function and evidence of pulmonary hypertension (TR V_{max}, RV outflow acceleration time).
LA volume (as a sign of chronically high LV filling pressures).
IVC size and response to respiration.
Valve appearance and function.
Constriction checklist (Tables 17.5 and 17.6 on pages 196, 197) if restrictive LV filling with normal LV ejection fraction.

Table 20.3 **Checklist in stroke, TIA or peripheral embolism[1]**

LV global hypokinesis, aneurysm, or large regional wall motion abnormality.
LV cardiomyopathy (DCM, HCM, non-compaction).
Signs of hypertension (see Table 20.4) as the underlying cause.
Mitral valve disease: stenosis > regurgitation.
Evidence of endocarditis.
Masses intracardiac tumours (e.g. LA myxoma, sarcoma), LV thrombus, LA or LAA thrombus,* fibroelastoma.
ASD or patent foramen ovale (bubble study according to clinical indications usually in patients aged < 50).
Aortic arch and ascending aortic atheroma.
Evidence of aortic dissection: dilated aorta, dissection flap (rarely presents without chest pain).
Atrial fibrillation or flutter (may occasionally be first diagnosed on TTE, especially if paroxysmal).

* Will usually require TOE, CT, or CMR.

Table 20.4 **Checklist in hypertension**

LV size and thickness (subaortic septal bulge may be an early sign but is also seen in normotensive elderly people).
LV systolic and diastolic function.
LA volume.
Aortic dimensions (sinus, sinotubular junction, and ascending aorta).
Coarctation in the young.
Aortic valve thickening and competence.

Table 20.5 **Checklist after arrhythmia**

After ventricular tachycardia[2]
LV size, wall thickness, and systolic function (especially evidence of aneurysm or any other wall motion abnormality).
RV size and systolic function (evidence of ARVC/D [see page 75]).
Severe valve disease.
Mitral annular dysjunction.
Atrial fibrillation or flutter
LA volume and RA area. LA thrombus?
Interatrial septum (check for ASD).
LV size and systolic and diastolic function.
RV size and function and PA pressure.
Mitral valve appearance and function.

Table 20.6 **Checklist in cocaine[3]**

Acute
Wall motion abnormality (myocardial infarction)
Generalised LV hypokinesis (myocarditis)
Aortic dissection
Long-term use
Dilated LV
LV hypertrophy
Evidence of endocarditis

Table 20.7 **Checklist in HIV[4]**

Dilated LV
LV systolic dysfunction (commonly mild, less commonly severe)
LV diastolic dysfunction
Pulmonary hypertension
Pericardial effusion
Evidence of endocarditis (increased susceptibility to infection)
Pericardial thickening and malignancy (e.g. Kaposi's sarcoma, non-Hodgkin's lymphoma)

Table 20.8 **TTE abnormalities in neuromuscular disorders**[5-8]

Duchenne muscular dystrophy	Regional wall motion abnormalities, usually inferolateral, from age 10 yr (mid-wall fibrosis may show on CMR even with normal TTE). By 18 yr, nearly all have cardiomyopathies, usually dilated. Some have LV hypertrophy. Pulmonary hypertension and RV dysfunction (secondary to respiratory failure) almost universal.
Becker muscular dystrophy	Dilated cardiomyopathy; usually begins in the inferolateral wall. ~40% have DCM on TTE by age 30 yr. CMR may show inferolateral mid-wall fibrosis, even with normal TTE.
Facioscapulohumeral muscular dystrophy	Cardiomyopathy rare.
Myotonic dystrophy	LV hypertrophy in ~20%. LV dilatation and systolic dysfunction in ~14%. CMR: Dilatation, hypertrophy, and reduced LV ejection fraction detected earlier than TTE.
Emery-Dreifuss muscular dystrophy	DCM moderately common. Unlike Duchenne and Becker, early disease not associated with fibrosis on CMR.
Limb girdle dystrophy (genetically and clinically heterogenous disorders with proximal muscular weakness)	Cardiac involvement is disease- and genetics-specific and can result in DCM with RV and LV fatty infiltration: • Type 2A and 2B most common: DCM rare. • Types 2C–2F: DCM common. • The lamin mutation subgroup can have diastolic dysfunction and mid-wall fibrosis of the basal infero-septum on CMR.
Friedrich's ataxia	LV hypertrophy: Concentric > asymmetric. Reduced LV ejection fraction in more severe cases. CMR may show inferolateral mid-wall fibrosis.
Mitochondrial cardiomyopathies	
MELAS/MERRF	HCM in 50%, DCM, and non-compaction also seen. Restrictive cardiomyopathy rare.
Kearns–Sayre	DCM uncommon. May have mitral and tricuspid prolapse.

Abbreviations: CMR, cardiac magnetic resonance scan; DCM, dilated cardiomyopathy; HCM, hypertrophic cardiomyopathy.

Table 20.9 Checklist in systemic inflammatory diseases[9]

Systemic lupus erythematosus (SLE)	LV dysfunction secondary to myocarditis. Generalised valve thickening and vegetations (mitral and aortic most commonly affected) with regurgitation (stenosis very rare). Pulmonary hypertension. Pericardial effusion (tamponade uncommon).
Primary antiphospholipid syndrome	Generalised valve thickening and vegetations (mitral and aortic most commonly affected) with regurgitation (stenosis very rare). Right-sided thrombus. Pulmonary hypertension. LV dysfunction (secondary to systemic hypertension or coronary disease).
Rheumatoid arthritis	Nodules typically at base of leaflets. Valve thickening commonly mild and focal but may be diffuse.
Ankylosing spondylitis	Aortic root dilatation with thickening and fibrosis of the base of the aortic cusps and anterior mitral leaflet.
Granulomatosis with polyangiitis	Aortic valve vegetations with regurgitation. Pericarditis. LV systolic dysfunction. Aortic aneurysms.
Eosinophilic granulomatosis with polyangiitis	Myocarditis common. Pericardial effusion.
Systemic sclerosis (scleroderma)	Myocardial fibrosis leading to diastolic > systolic LV dysfunction. Pulmonary hypertension and RV failure (secondary to lung fibrosis). Pericardial effusion (c40%). Aortic or mitral valve thickening (c10%).
Polymyositis/dermatomyositis	LV diastolic dysfunction (40%). Pulmonary hypertension (interstitial lung disease).
Mixed connective tissue disease	Pulmonary hypertension.
Sjögren's syndrome	Cardiac involvement uncommon. Pulmonary hypertension (secondary to lung involvement).
Behçet's disease	Myocarditis. RA and RV thrombus. Pulmonary artery aneurysms.

(Continued)

Table 20.9 **Checklist in systemic inflammatory diseases** (Continued)

Cogan's disease	Aortic dilatation and aortic regurgitation.
Sarcoidosis	See Table 7.4, page 64.
Takayasu's arteritis	Aortic dilatation with secondary aortic regurgitation. Pulmonary artery dilatation. Pulmonary stenosis. Fistulae between pulmonary artery and coronary or bronchial arteries or aorta. Subclinical myocardial involvement.
Giant cell arteritis	Thoracic aortic aneurysm.
Polyarteritis nodosa	DCM.
Microscopic polyangiitis	Heart failure. Pericarditis.
Kawasaki disease	Myocardial infarction. Myocarditis and pericarditis acutely.

Table 20.10 **Checklist in hypereosinophilia, Loeffler's endocarditis, endomyocardial fibrosis**[10]

LV or RV apical cavity obliteration by thrombus and fibrosis (Figure 7.2)
Hyperdense endocardium
Restrictive cardiomyopathy
Fibrous attachment of tricuspid and mitral valves with mitral and tricuspid regurgitation

Table 20.11 **Checklist in drug treatment with dopamine agonists (pergolide and cabergoline), appetite suppressants (fenfluramine and dexfenfluramine), and the weight loss agent benfluorex**[11]

More commonly affecting mitral and aortic valves: • Leaflet thickening, restriction, and regurgitation (stenosis uncommon). • Chordal thickening and shortening. • First sign may be increased tenting height of the mitral valve. • Thickening affects the whole leaflet.

Note: Abnormalities almost never seen with low-dose use in microprolactinoma.

Table 20.12 **Checklist in radiation**[12]

Valve disease	Aortic and mitral valve thickening, fibrosis, shortening, and calcification Regurgitation more common than stenosis Incidence 6% at 20 years after irradiation
LV dysfunction	Diffuse myocardial fibrosis Initially systolic dysfunction, later restrictive cardiomyopathy
Coronary disease	Accelerated coronary disease Regional wall motion abnormalities
Pericardial disease	Chronic pericarditis: pericardial thickening, adhesions, effusion Pericardial constriction: Incidence 4–20%, depending on dose and concomitant use of chemotherapy

References

1. Cohen A, Donal E, Delgado V, et al. EACVI Recommendations on cardiovascular imaging for the detection of embolic sources: Endorsed by the Canadian Society of Echocardiography. Eur Heart J Cardiovasc Imaging 2021;22(6):E24–57.
2. Dejgaard LA, Skjølsvik ET, Lie ØH, et al. The mitral annulus disjunction arrhythmic syndrome. J Am Coll Cardiol 2018;72(14):1600–9.
3. Missouris CG, Swift PA & Singer DR. Cocaine use and acute left ventricular dysfunction. Lancet 2001;357(9268):1586.
4. Reinsch N, Kahlert P, Esser S, et al. Echocardiographic findings and abnormalities in HIV-infected patients: Results from a large, prospective, multicenter HIV-heart study. Am J Cardiovasc Dis 2011;1(2):176–84.
5. Verhaert D, Richards K, Rafael-Fortney JA, et al. Cardiac involvement in patients with muscular dystrophies: Magnetic resonance imaging phenotype and genotypic considerations. Circ Cardiovasc Imaging 2011;4(1):67–76.
6. Beynon RP & Ray SG. Cardiac involvement in muscular dystrophies. Q J Med 2008;101(5):337–44.
7. Weidemann F, Rummey C, Bijnens B, et al. The heart in Friedreich ataxia: Definition of cardiomyopathy, disease severity, and correlation with neurological symptoms. Circulation 2012;125(13):1626–34.
8. El-Hattab AW & Scaglia F. Mitochondrial cardiomyopathies. Front Cardiovasc Med 2016;3(25):1–9.
9. Roldan CA. Valvular and coronary heart disease in systemic inflammatory diseases. Heart 2008;94(8):1089–1.

10. Mankad R, Bonnichsen C & Mankad S. Hypereosinophilic syndrome: Cardiac diagnosis and management. Heart 2016;102(2):100–6.
11. Andrejak M & Tribouilloy C. Drug-induced valvular heart disease: An update. Arch Cardiovasc Dis 2013;106(5):333–9.
12. Lancellotti P, Nkomo VT, Badano LP, et al. Expert consensus for multi-modality imaging evaluation of cardiovascular complications of radiotherapy in adults: A report from the European Association of Cardiovascular Imaging and the American Society of Echocardiography. Eur Hear J 2013;14(8):721–40.

Appendices

Left Ventricle

Cardiac Resynchronisation

1. **Patient selection**
   - The decision for CRT[1]:
     - NYHA class III and IV unresponsive to maximal heart failure therapy
     - LVEF ≤35%
     - ECG QRS >120 ms and ideally >150 ms[2]
   - Use contrast agents to enhance endocardial delineation if the image quality is suboptimal.
   - Use 3D when image quality is good and staff have expertise in 3D data acquisition and processing. Ideally, use vendor-neutral analysis software.

2. **Cardiac resynchronisation optimisation**
   - Echocardiographic optimisation is not routine but should be used for patients with refractory symptoms. There is no consensus, but a guide is:

   2.1 Perform a baseline TTE to assess LV remodelling.
   - LV dimensions, volumes, and global and regional systolic function.
   - Assess MR, TR severity, and PA systolic pressure.
   - Compare measurements with the pre-CRT values and report changes.
   - Check that Bi-V pacing >90%. If not, do not continue optimisation. The pacing physiologist will optimise pacemaker settings.

   2.2 Start with AV delay optimisation (cannot perform if patient in AF).

Mitral valve filling time and aortic valve VTI method:
   - Annotate pacemaker baseline settings on the screen (mode, base rate, AV delay). Set up VV delay at 0–4 ms (both ventricles activate at the same time).
   - Record PW Doppler of mitral valve inflow and optimise trace for best visualisation of A wave and opening and closing artefacts.
   - Measure diastolic filling ratio (LV filling time/RR interval) at baseline. Significant atrioventricular dyssynchrony is assumed if this ratio is <40%.
   - Record aortic valve CW Doppler and optimise trace for best visualisation of opening and closing artefacts. Measure baseline VTI_{aortic} (or $VTI_{subaortic}$ if there is aortic stenosis).

- Ask a pacing physiologist to change the AV delay in incremental steps of 10–20 ms within the range from 80 to 180 ms. Annotate AV delay on the screen and measure diastolic filling ratio and VTI $_{aortic}$ at multiple settings.
- With longer AV delays, check you have not lost Bi-V pacing. If so, come down to the longest AV delay that still enables Bi-V pacing.
- Compare measurements and select the AV delay with the highest diastolic filling ratio and VTI$_{aortic}$ values.

Alternative proposed method—truncation of A wave method:

- Assess mitral valve pulsed Doppler inflow A wave[3]:
  - When A wave is blunted, the AV delay is too short.
  - When E and A partially overlap or diastolic MR appears, the AV delay is too long.
- Choose the AV delay with the best developed A wave without shortening the A deceleration time, and with the least mitral regurgitation.

2.3 Optimise interventricular delay:

- Set to the optimal AV delay.
- Select different VV delays and annotate them on the screen:
  - Both ventricles activated at the same time—baseline.
  - The RV activated earlier than the left (e.g. 30 ms and 50 ms).
  - The LV activated earlier than the right (e.g. 30 ms and 50 ms).
- Measure VTI$_{aortic}$ (VTI$_{subaortic}$ if there is aortic stenosis) at different settings and choose the sequence with the highest value.

CHECKLIST FOR REPORTING CRT OPTIMISATION:

1. Device implantation date.
2. Changes in symptoms after device implantation.
3. Optimal AV delay (ms).
4. Optimal VV delay (ms).
5. Parameters of LV remodelling and changes when compared to pre-implantation data.
6. MR severity.
7. TR severity and PA systolic pressure.

Critical Care Monitoring

- Suitability for ECMO (Table A.1)
- Monitoring ECMO (Table A.2)

- Weaning from ECMO (Table A.3)
- Checklist for ventricular assist device (Table A.4)
- Intra-aortic balloon pump (Table A.5)

Table A.1 Suitability for ECMO (extracorporeal membrane oxygenation)

Reversible pathology avoiding ECMO
Pericardial tamponade
Surgically correctible valve disease
Indications for venovenous ECMO
Respiratory failure
Needs venoarterial rather than venovenous ECMO
Severe PA hypertension (mean PA pressure >50 mmHg)
Severe LV impairment
Severe valve disease
Absolute contraindication for venoarterial ECMO
Severe aortic regurgitation
Unrepaired aortic dissection
Widespread LV scarring
Use peripheral rather than central lines
Aortic atheroma
ASD, large PFO, atrial septal aneurysm

Table A.2 Echocardiographic monitoring for ECMO[5-7]

Confirm correct position of cannulae.
Access cannula near mouth of IVC.
Return cannula in mid-RA clear of interatrial septum and tricuspid valve.
Incorrect positions include the coronary sinus or RV or LA via a PFO.
General
LV and RV function.
Grade of any mitral regurgitation.
Aortic valve opening.
Pericardial fluid.

(Continued)

Table A.2 **Echocardiographic monitoring for ECMO**[5-7] (Continued)

Complications
Cannula displacement.
Cannula thrombosis.
Obstruction of veins or arteries.
LV thrombus.
Tamponade.
Pulmonary embolism.
Hypoxia from recirculation.

Table A.3 **Echocardiographic features supporting weaning from VA ECMO with flow reduction to <1.5 L/min**[5-7]

LVEF >20–25% and ideally >35%
VTI$_{lvot}$ ≥10 cm
Tissue Doppler peak systolic velocity ≥6 cm/s
Non-dilated LV
No cardiac tamponade

Table A.4 **Checklist for temporary ventricular assist device**[8, 9]

Before insertion
LV size and function (diastolic volume <120 mL may limit effectiveness)
RV size and function
Grade of mitral and tricuspid regurgitation
Contraindications
Aortic pathology (dissection, abdominal or thoracic aortic aneurysm)
LV apical thrombus
Aortic stenosis or regurgitation
Small LV cavity (e.g. HCM)
ASD
Severe RV dysfunction (RV area change <20% may develop RV failure)
Severe pulmonary hypertension (systolic pressure >50 mmHg)

At insertion
Correct position (parasternal or apical long-axis view): • Inlet area 40–45 mm below aortic valve. • Catheter angled towards the LV apex. • Catheter not curled up or obstructing the mitral valve or with the tip in the papillary muscle area.
Colour Doppler mosaic flow pattern of the exit stream above the sinus of Valsalva.
Optimise LV filling: • Maximise E wave velocity and VTI_{mitral}. • Septal shift to right means pump flow too low. • Septal shift to left means pump flow too high.
Exclude right-to-left atrial shunting.
Monitoring
Verify position of catheter.
Verify outflow mosaic pattern above the sinus of Valsalva.
Confirm permanently closed aortic and pulmonary valves.
LV and RV systolic function: • Echo-guided increase in pump speed for LV failure. • Echo-guided decrease in pump speed for RV failure.
Ventricular unloading (transmitral E wave).
PA pressure.
Grade of mitral regurgitation.
Check for pericardial effusion.
Exclude LV thrombus.

Table A.5 **Checklist for intra-aortic balloon pump**

Contraindications
Moderate or severe aortic regurgitation
Aortic pathology (severe atheroma, dissection, abdominal aneurysm)
Monitoring
Correct position (tip at junction of arch and descending thoracic aorta)
Change in $VTI_{subaortic}$ with augmentation
Leakage (bubbles in aorta)
Exclude pericardial effusion

Valve Disease

- Wilkins score (Table A.6)
- Duke criteria for diagnosing endocarditis (Table A.7)
- Normal ranges for prosthetic heart valves (Tables A.8–A.10)

Table A.6 **Wilkins score**[10]

Morphology	Score
Mobility	
Highly mobile, only tips restricted	1
Normal mobility of base and mid-leaflet	2
Valve moves forward in diastole mainly from the base	3
No or minimal movement	4
Leaflet thickening	
Near normal	1
Thickening mainly at tips	2
Thickening (5–8 mm) over the whole leaflet	3
Severe thickening (>8 mm) of whole leaflet	4
Subvalvar thickening	
Minimal, just below leaflets	1
Over one-third of the chords	2
Extending to the distal third of the chords	3
Extensive thickening and shortening of the whole chord	4
Calcification	
A single area of echogenicity	1
Scattered areas at leaflet margin	2
Echogenicity extending to midportion of leaflets	3
Extensive echogenicity over whole leaflet	4

Note: A total score ≤8 suggests a successful result, but the score has not been validated in a large population and does not assess some key points (Table 9.4, page 106).

Table A.7 **Modified Duke clinical criteria for infective endocarditis**[11]

Major—Microbiological	Major—Echocardiographic	Minor

1. Typical microorganisms consistent with IE from two separate sets of blood cultures: for example, oral streptococci, *Streptococcus bovis* group, HACEK group, *S. aureus* or community-acquired enterococci (in the absence of a primary focus)
 	
or
 	
2. Microorganisms consistent with IE from persistently positive blood cultures: at least 2 positive blood cultures taken 12 h apart or all 3 or a majority of 4 separate blood cultures (1 hr between 1st and last samples)
 	
or
 	
3. Single positive blood culture for *Coxiella burnetti* or phase 1 IgG antibody titre >1:800
	1. Vegetations
	
	or
	
	2. Abscess
	
	or
	
	3. Dehiscence of a prosthetic valve
	
	or
	
	4. Perforation of a valve
	
	or
	
	5. Fistula formation
	
	or PET positive for prosthetic valve or abscess on CT
		1. At risk heart condition, IVDU
		2. Fever > 38°C
		3. Vascular phenomena
		  • Emboli
		  • Septic pulmonary infarcts
		  • Intracranial haemorrhage
		  • Mycotic aneurysm
		4. Immunologic phenomena
		  • Glomerulonephritis
		  • Rheumatoid factor
		  • Roth spots, etc.
		5. Microbiology other than major criteria

Normal values for prosthetic heart valves: mean (standard deviation)

(Table A.8–Table A.10)[12–14]

- The Hatle formula for mitral orifice area (220/pressure half-time) is not valid in normally functioning mitral prostheses.
- Doppler results are broadly similar for valves sharing a similar design. For simplicity, results for one design in each category is given with a list of other valve designs for which data exist.
- Sizing conventions vary, so it is possible that a given label size for a valve not on the list may not be equivalent to those that are. A change on serial studies is more revealing than a single measurement, and the TTE must be interpreted in the clinical context.

Table A.8 **Aortic position—biological valves, mean (SD) values**

Stented Porcine—Carpentier-Edwards standard as example (values similar for Carpentier-Edwards supra-annular, Intact, Hancock I and II and Mosaic, Biocor, Epic)			
	V_{max} m/s	Peak ΔP mmHg	Mean ΔP mmHg	EOA cm^2
19 mm		43.5 (12.7)	25.6 (8.0)	0.9 (0.2)
21 mm	2.8 (0.5)	27.2 (7.6)	17.3 (6.2)	1.5 (0.3)
23 mm	2.8 (0.7)	28.9 (7.5)	16.1 (6.2)	1.7 (0.5)
25 mm	2.6 (0.6)	24.0 (7.1)	12.9 (4.6)	1.9 (0.5)
27 mm	2.5 (0.5)	22.1 (8.2)	12.1 (5.5)	2.3 (0.6)
29 mm	2.4 (0.4)		9.9 (2.9)	2.8 (0.5)
Stented Bovine Pericardial—Edwards Perimount as example (similar for Mitroflow, Edwards Pericardial, Labcor-Santiago, Mitroflow)			
19 mm	2.8 (0.1)	32.5 (8.5)	19.5 (5.5)	1.3 (0.2)
21 mm	2.6 (0.4)	24.9 (7.7)	13.8 (4.0)	1.3 (0.3)
23 mm	2.3 (0.5)	19.9 (7.4)	11.5 (3.9)	1.6 (0.3)
25 mm	2.0 (0.3)	16.5 (7.8)	10.7 (3.8)	1.6 (0.4)
27 mm		12.8 (5.4)	4.8 (2.2)	2.0 (0.4)
Homograft			
22 mm	1.7 (0.3)		5.8 (3.2)	2.0 (0.6)
26 mm	1.4 (0.6)		6.8 (2.9)	2.4 (0.7)
Stentless—St Jude Toronto (similar to Prima)			
21 mm		22.6 (14.5)	10.7 (7.2)	1.3 (0.6)
23 mm		16.2 (9.0)	8.2 (4.7)	1.6 (0.6)
25 mm		12.7 (8.2)	6.3 (4.1)	1.8 (0.5)
27 mm		10.1 (5.8)	5.0 (2.9)	2.0 (0.3)
29 mm		7.7 (4.4)	4.1 (2.4)	2.4 (0.6)

Table A.9 **Aortic position—mechanical, mean (SD) values**

Single tilting disk
Medtronic-Hall (similar values Bjork-Shiley monostrut and CC, Omnicarbon, and Omniscience)

	V_{max} m/s	Peak ΔP mmHg	Mean ΔP mmHg	EOA cm²
20 mm	2.9 (0.4)	34.4 (13.1)	17.1 (5.3)	1.2 (0.5)
21 mm	2.4 (0.4)	26.9 (10.5)	14.1 (5.9)	1.1 (0.2)
23 mm	2.4 (0.6)	26.9 (8.9)	13.5 (4.8)	1.4 (0.4)
25 mm	2.3 (0.5)	17.1 (7.0)	9.5 (4.3)	1.5 (0.5)
27 mm	2.1 (0.5)	18.9 (9.7)	8.7 (5.6)	1.9 (0.2)

Bileaflet mechanical
Intrannular—St Jude standard (similar Carbomedics standard, Edwards Mira, ATS, Sorin Bicarbon)

	V_{max} m/s	Peak ΔP mmHg	Mean ΔP mmHg	EOA cm²
19 mm	2.9 (0.5)	35.2 (11.2)	19.0 (6.3)	1.0 (0.2)
21 mm	2.6 (0.5)	28.3 (10.0)	15.8 (5.7)	1.3 (0.3)
23 mm	2.6 (0.4)	25.3 (7.9)	13.8 (5.3)	1.6 (0.4)
25 mm	2.4 (0.5)	22.6 (7.7)	12.7 (5.1)	1.9 (0.5)
27 mm	2.2 (0.4)	19.9 (7.6)	11.2 (4.8)	2.4 (0.6)
29 mm	2.0 (0.1)	17.7 (6.4)	9.9 (2.9)	2.8 (0.6)

Intra-annular modified cuff or partially supra-annular—On-X (similar St Jude Regent, St Jude HP, Carbomedics Reduced cuff, Medtronic Advantage)

	V_{max} m/s	Peak ΔP mmHg	Mean ΔP mmHg	EOA cm²
19 mm		21.3 (10.8)	11.8 (3.4)	1.5 (0.2)
21 mm		16.4 (5.9)	9.9 (3.6)	1.7 (0.4)
23 mm		15.9 (6.4)	8.6 (3.4)	1.9 (0.6)
25 mm		16.5 (10.2)	6.9 (4.3)	2.4 (0.6)

Supra-annular—Carbomedics TopHat

	V_{max} m/s	Peak ΔP mmHg	Mean ΔP mmHg	EOA cm²
21mm	2.6 (0.4)	30.2 (10.9)	14.9 (5.4)	1.2 (0.3)
23mm	2.4 (0.6)	24.2 (7.6)	12.5 (4.4)	1.4 (0.4)
25mm			9.5 (2.9)	1.6 (0.3)

(Continued)

Table A.9 **Aortic position—mechanical, mean (SD) values** (Continued)

Ball and cage—Starr-Edwards				
	V_{max} m/s	Peak ΔP mmHg	Mean ΔP mmHg	EOA cm²
23 mm	3.4 (0.6)	32.6 (12.8)	22.0 (9.0)	1.1 (0.2)
24 mm	3.6 (0.5)	34.1 (10.3)	22.1 (7.5)	1.1 (0.3)
26 mm	3.0 (0.2)	31.8 (9.0)	19.7 (6.1)	
27 mm		30.8 (6.3)	18.5 (3.7)	
29 mm		29.3 (9.3)	16.3 (5.5)	

Table A.10 **Mitral position, mean (SD) values**

Stented Porcine—Carpentier-Edwards (similar Intact, Hancock)			
	V_{max} m/s	Mean ΔP mmHg	EOA cm²
25 mm	1.5 (0.4)		
27 mm		6.0 (2.0)	1.8 (0.5)
29 mm	1.5 (0.3)	4.7 (2.0)	1.9 (0.5)
31 mm	1.5 (0.3)	4.5 (2.0)	2.6 (0.5)
33 mm	1.4 (0.2)	5.4 (4.0)	2.6 (0.5)
Pericardial—Edwards Perimount (similar Labcor-Santiago, Hancock pericardial)			
25 mm	1.4 (0.2)	4.9 (1.1)	1.6 (0.4)
27 mm	1.3 (0.2)	3.2 (0.8)	1.8 (0.4)
29 mm	1.4 (0.2)	3.2 (0.6)	2.1 (0.5)
31 mm	1.3 (0.1)	2.7 (0.4)	
Single tilting disc—Bjork-Shiley monostrut (similar Omnicarbon)			
25 mm	1.8 (0.3)	5.6 (2.3)	
27 mm	1.7 (0.4)	4.5 (2.2)	
29 mm	1.6 (0.3)	4.3 (1.6)	
31 mm	1.7 (0.3)	4.9 (1.6)	
33 mm	1.3 (0.3)		

Bileaflet—Carbomedics (similar St Jude)			
25 mm	1.6 (0.2)	4.3 (0.7)	1.5 (0.3)
27 mm	1.6 (0.3)	3.7 (1.5)	1.7 (0.4)
29 mm	1.8 (0.3)	3.7 (1.3)	1.8 (0.4)
31 mm	1.6 (0.4)	3.3 (1.1)	2.0 (0.5)
33 mm	1.4 (0.3)	3.4 (1.5)	2.0 (0.5)
OnX			
All sizes			2.2 (0.9)
Caged ball—Starr-Edwards			
28 mm	1.8 (0.2)	7.0 (2.8)	
30 mm	1.8 (0.2)	7.0 (2.5)	
32 mm	1.9 (0.4)	5.1 (2.5)	

Aorta

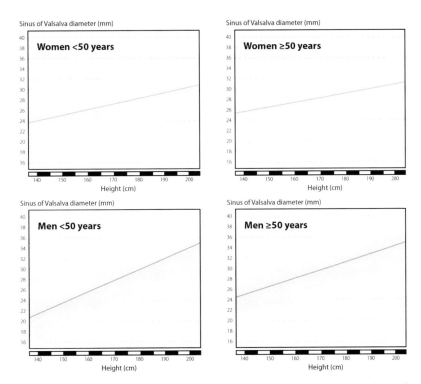

Figure A.1 **Nomograms for sinus of Valsalva diameter against height in men and women aged above and below 50. (**Redrawn from data in [15], with permission of Oxford University Press.)

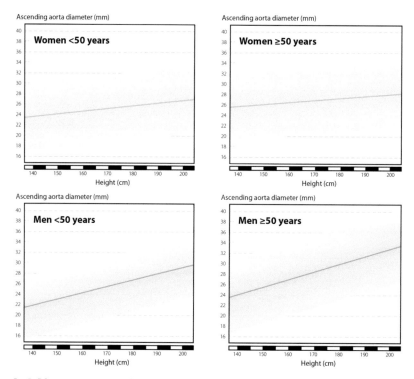

Nomograms for ascending aortic diameter against height in men and women aged above and below 50. (Redrawn from data in [15], with permission of Oxford University Press.)

Summary of Formulae

1. Bernoulli equation

This equates potential and kinetic energy up- and downstream from a stenosis. The modified formula is used in two forms:

Short modified Bernoulli equation $\Delta P \text{ (mmHg)} = 4\,v_2^2$
Long modified Bernoulli equation $\Delta P \text{ (mmHg)} = 4\,(v_2^2 - v_1^2)$

where ΔP is transvalvar pressure difference, v_1 is subvalvar velocity, and v_2 is transvalvar velocity.

The short form can be used when subvalvar is much less than transvalvar velocity, for example, mitral stenosis, moderate or severe aortic stenosis ($V_2 > 3.0$ m/s), but not mild aortic stenosis or normally functioning replacement valves.

2. Continuity equation

$$EOA \ (cm^2) = CSA \times VTI_{subaortic} / VTI_{ao}$$

where *EOA* is effective orifice area, *CSA* is cross-sectional area of the LV outflow tract, $VTI_{subaortic}$ and VTI_{ao} are subaortic and transaortic systolic velocity time integral. For prosthetic mitral valves, the velocity time integral of the transmitral signal can be substituted for VTI_{ao}.

3. Pressure half-time estimation of mitral orifice area

$$MOA \ (cm^2) = 220/T1/2$$

where *MOA* is effective mitral orifice area and *T1/2* is pressure half-time in ms. This formula should only be used in moderate or severe stenosis. It is not valid in normally functioning replacement valves. The pressure half-time is shortened in mitral stenosis if there is significant MR or AR.

4. Stroke volume and cardiac output

$$SV \ (mL) = CSA \times VTI_{subaortic}$$

where *CSA* is cross-sectional area of the left ventricular outflow tract (in cm^2) and $VTI_{subaortic}$ is subaortic velocity integral (in cm).

$$Cardiac \ output \ (mL/min) = SV \times heart \ rate$$

5. Flow

$$Flow \ (mL/s) = CSA \times VTI_{subaortic} \times 1{,}000/SET$$

where *CSA* is cross-sectional area of the LV outflow tract (in cm^2), $VTI_{subaortic}$ is subaortic velocity integral (in cm), and *SET* is systolic ejection time (from opening to closing artefact of the aortic signal) (in ms).

A number of formulae, 6–10, are sometimes used in research.

6. Energy Loss Index (ELI)

$$ELI \ (cm^2/m^2) = [(EOA.A_{STJ})/(A_{STJ}-EOA)]/BSA$$

where *EOA* is effective orifice area in cm^2 using the continuity equation (equation 2), A_{STJ} is cross-sectional area of the aorta at the level of the sinotubular junction, and *BSA* is body surface area in m^2.
ELI <0.6 cm^2/m^2 is a common cut point for severe AS.

7. Total VA (ventriculo-aortic) impedance

$$\Sigma va\ (mmHg/mL/m^2) = (mean\ \Delta P + SBP)/SVI$$

where mean ΔP is recovered pressure (equation 8) in mmHg, *SBP* is systolic blood pressure in mmHg, and *SVI* is stroke volume indexed to BSA in mL/m².

8. Recovered mean pressure gradient in aortic stenosis

$$Recovered\ \Delta P\ (mmHg) = 4v_2^2.2(EOA/A_{STJ})(1-EOA/A_{STJ})$$

where *v* is the transaortic V_{max} in m/s, *EOA* is the effective orifice area in cm², and A_{STJ} is the area of the aorta at the sinotubular junction in cm².

9. Stroke work loss

$$SWL(\%) = 100.mean\ \Delta P/(mean\ \Delta P + SBP)$$

where ΔP is mean gradient from the transaortic continuous wave signal in mmHg and *SBP* is systolic blood pressure in mmHg.

10. Systemic vascular resistance

$$Systemic\ vascular\ resistance\ (dyne.sec/cm^5) = (mean\ arterial\ pressure \times 80)/cardiac\ output$$

where *mean arterial pressure* is in mmHg and *cardiac output* is in L/min. Normal is 800–1,200 dyne.sec/cm⁵.

Shunt Calculation

Table A.11 Chamber volume load and levels for shunt calculation

		Level for shunt calculation	
	Loaded chamber	Downstream	Upstream
ASD	RV	Pulmonary artery	LV outflow
VSD	LV	Pulmonary artery	LV outflow
PDA	LV	LV outflow	Pulmonary valve

- The stroke volume is calculated for the aortic valve (equation 4) and then for the pulmonary valve using the diameter at the pulmonary annulus and the VTI calculated with the pulsed sample at the level of the annulus.
- If the annulus cannot be imaged reliably, the diameter of the pulmonary artery and the level for velocity recording should be taken at a downstream point, where imaging is possible.
- The shunt is then the ratio of the downstream to the upstream stroke volume (Table A.11).

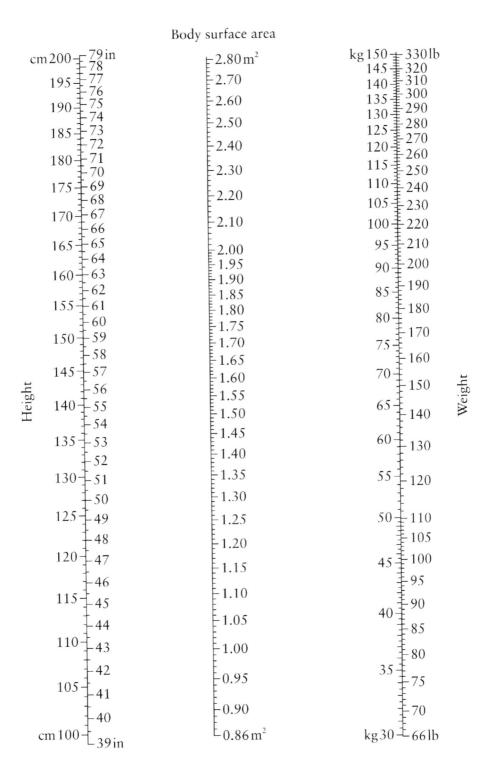

Body surface area

Figure A.3 Body surface nomogram. Put a straight edge against the patient's height and weight and read off the body surface area on the middle column.

References

1. Chung ES, Leon AR, Tavazzi L, et al. Heart failure: Results of the predictors of response to CRT (PROSPECT) trial. Circulation 2008;117:2608–16.
2. Gorcsan III J & Delgado-Montero A. The current role of echocardiography in cardiac resynchronisation therapy. Hjerteforum 2015;1(28):34–42.
3. EACVI 3D. Echocardiography Box: Echo parameters in CRT patients' selection. https://www.escardio.org/Education/Practice-Tools/EACVI-toolboxes/3D-Echo/echo-parameters-in-crt-patients-selection.
4. Kuznetsov VA, Soldatova AM, Kaprzak DV & Melnikov NN. Echocardiographic markers of dyssynchrony as predictors of super-response to cardiac resynchronisation therapy—A pilot study. Cardiovasc Ultrasound 2018;16(1):24.
5. Kapoor PM. Echocardiography in extra corporeal membrane oxygenation. Ann Card Anaesth 2017;20(Suppl 1):S1–3
6. Bailleul C & Aissaoui N. Role of echocardiography in the management of veno-arterial extra-corporeal membrane oxygenation. J Emerg Critic Care Medicine 2019;3:25. doi:10.21037/jeccm.2019.05.03
7. Ictor K, Barrett NA, Gillon S, et al. Critical care echo rounds: Extracorporeal membrane oxygenation. Echo Res Pract 2015;2:D1–1.
8. Mehrotra AK, Shah D, Sugeng L & Jolly N. Echocardiography for percutaneous heart pumps. J Am Coll Cardiol CVI 2009;2:1332–3.
9. Catena E, Milazzo F, Merli M, et al. Echocardiographic evaluation of patients receiving a new left ventricular assist device: The Impella Recover 100. Eur J Echo 2004;5:430–7.
10. Wilkins GT, Weyman AE, Abascal VM, Block PC & Palacios IF. Percutaneous balloon dilatation of the mitral valve: An analysis of echocardiographic variables related to outcome and the mechanism of dilatation. Brit Heart J 1988;60:299–308.
11. Habib G, Lancellotti P, Antunes MJ, et al. 2015 ESC Guidelines for the management of infective endocarditis. Europ Heart J 2015;36:3075–128.
12. Rajani R, Mukherjee D & Chambers J. Doppler echocardiography in normally functioning replacement aortic valves: A literature review. J Heart Valve Dis 2007;16:519–35.
13. Rosenhek R, Binder T, Maurer G & Baumgartner H. Normal values for Doppler echocardiographic assessment of heart valve prostheses. J Am Soc Echo 2003;16(11):1116–27.
14. Pibarot P & Dumesnil JG. Prosthetic heart valves: Selection of the optimal prosthesis and long-term management. Circulation 2009;119:1034–48.
15. Saura D, Dulgheru R, Caballero L, et al. Two-dimensional transthoracic echocardiographic normal reference ranges for proximal aorta dimensions: Results from the EACVI NORRE study. Eur Heart J CVI 2017;18(2):167–79.

Index

Note: Page numbers in **bold** indicate a table and page numbers in *italics* indicate a figure on the corresponding page.